Dark Calories and Toxic Oils Detox for Healthy Healing

Exposing the Dark Side of Seed Oils and Vegetable Oils to Find Your Path to Wellness

Dr. Charlotte Jay

CONTENTS

CONTENTS 3

ABSTRACT 9

INTRODUCTION 11

    The Hidden Crisis in Our Food 11

    Understanding Dark Calories 16

PART I: THE DARK SIDE OF SEED OILS AND VEGETABLE OILS 23

    1)   THE RISE OF VEGETABLE OILS 24

        Historical Background 24

        The Influence of Big Industry 30

        Evolution of Dietary Guidelines 35

2) UNMASKING DARK CALORIES 41

   Defining Dark Calories 41

   The Biochemistry of Harmful Oils................................46

   How Dark Calories Affect Our Bodies........................53

3) HEALTH IMPACTS OF SEED AND VEGETABLE OILS 61

   Chronic inflammation...61

   Oxidative Stress and Cellular Damage.......................64

   Metabolic disorders and obesity.................................67

   Mental Health and Cognitive Function.....................69

4) THE DECEPTION OF 'HEALTHY' OILS.................73

   Myths vs. Facts...73

   Marketing Tactics and Misleading Health Claims .76

   Financial Interests and Industry Influence..............78

PART II: DETOXING FROM TOXIC OILS..............................81

5) UNDERSTANDING DETOXIFICATION 82

   The Body's Natural Detox Processes........................82

   The Role of Diet in Detoxification................................84

Common Detox Myths and Misconceptions.............87

6) ELIMINATING TOXIC OILS FROM YOUR DIET 91

Identifying Hidden Sources of Seed and Vegetable Oils 91

Reading Labels and Understanding Ingredients....92

Practical Tips for Avoidance at Aome and Eating Out................94

7) HEALTHY OIL ALTERNATIVES 98

Benefits of Olive Oil, Coconut Oil, and Other Healthy Fats 98

Incorporating nut and fruit oils................100

Cooking Techniques and Recipes Using Healthy Oils 103

8) SUPPLEMENTATION AND NUTRITIONAL SUPPORT 107

Essential Nutrients for Recovery................107

Antioxidant-Rich Foods and Supplements............110

Balancing Omega-3 and Omega-6 Fatty Acids.....113

PART III: HEALING AND RECOVERY................117

9) NUTRITIONAL STRATEGIES FOR RECOVERY 118

Anti-Inflammatory Foods 118

Rebuilding Cellular Health 122

Gut Health and Probiotics 125

10) REJUVENATING YOUR BODY 128

Supporting Antioxidant Levels 128

Detoxifying the Liver and Other Organs 130

Natural remedies and supplements 133

11) MENTAL AND EMOTIONAL WELL-BEING 136

Foods for Brain Health 136

Managing Mood and Energy Levels 139

Stress Reduction Techniques: 140

12) PHYSICAL FITNESS AND ACTIVITY 142

Exercise for Detox and Health 142

Building an Active Lifestyle 145

Yoga and Mindfulness Practices 147

13) CREATING A SUSTAINABLE HEALTHY LIFESTYLE 150

Long-term Dietary Changes 150

Meal Planning and Recipes 152

Building Healthy Eating Habits 155

PART IV: BEYOND THE KITCHEN 159

14) HOLISTIC APPROACHES TO WELLNESS 160

Integrating Mind, Body, and Spirit 160

Alternative Therapies and Practices 162

Sleep and Its Role in Healing 164

15) ADVOCACY AND AWARENESS 167

Educating Others About the Risks 167

Supporting Policy Changes for Healthier Food Standards 168

Community Involvement and Grassroots Movements 170

16) RESEARCH AND FUTURE DIRECTIONS 175

Emerging Studies and Trends 175

Innovations in Food Science and Nutrition 176

The Future of Dietary Guidelines 178

CONCLUSION 181

- APPENDICES 184
  - RESOURCES AND FURTHER READING 184
    - Recommended Books 184
    - Recommended Articles 185
    - Useful Websites and Organizations 186
  - GLOSSARY OF TERMS 188

ABSTRACT

"Dark Calories and Toxic Oils Detox for Healthy Healing" delves into the pervasive impact of seed oils and vegetable oils on human health, uncovering their role in chronic diseases such as cardiovascular conditions, metabolic disorders, and mental health issues. This comprehensive guide exposes the historical and industrial influences that shaped dietary guidelines promoting these oils as healthy, despite their detrimental effects.

The concept of "dark calories" is introduced to illuminate how these oils contribute to inflammation, oxidative stress, and cellular damage within the body. By exploring the biochemical mechanisms underlying their harm, readers gain insights into why these oils are detrimental to long-term health.

The book navigates through the deceptive marketing tactics and misleading health claims surrounding "healthy" oils, revealing the financial interests and industry influences driving their widespread consumption. Practical strategies are provided for identifying and eliminating hidden sources of these oils from everyday diets, empowering readers to make informed choices for their health.

Furthermore, the book emphasizes the importance of detoxifying from toxic oils and adopting healthier alternatives such as olive oil and coconut oil. It explores nutritional strategies for recovery, including the benefits of anti-inflammatory foods, antioxidant-rich diets, and balanced omega-3 and omega-6 fatty acids.

Beyond dietary considerations, "Dark Calories and Toxic Oils Detox for Healthy Healing" advocates for a holistic approach to wellness, integrating mind, body, and spirit. It discusses the role of gut health, probiotics, natural remedies, and stress reduction techniques in promoting overall well-being.

Looking forward, the book explores emerging studies, innovations in food science, and the future of dietary guidelines, emphasizing sustainable practices for personal and planetary health. It concludes with a call to action, urging advocacy for healthier food standards and community involvement to support holistic health initiatives.

INTRODUCTION

In "Dark Calories and Toxic Oils Detox for Healthy Healing," we embark on a journey to uncover the hidden dangers of commonly consumed oils and their profound impact on our health. This introduction sets the stage for a deep dive into the world of seed and vegetable oils, revealing their connection to chronic diseases and presenting actionable steps to detoxify our diets. By understanding the historical, industrial, and biochemical contexts, we can reclaim our health and embrace a more holistic approach to wellness.

The Hidden Crisis in Our Food

The modern food landscape is a battleground, a place where the war for our health is being fought quietly and often without our awareness. This crisis, deeply embedded in the very fabric of our dietary habits, has roots that stretch back several decades and branches that touch nearly every aspect of our lives. At its core, this crisis revolves around the pervasive use of seed oils and vegetable oils—substances that have been marketed as healthy alternatives but are, in fact, contributing to a wide array of chronic health issues.

The story begins in the early 20th century, a time when industrial advancements and agricultural innovations began to reshape the way food was produced and consumed. Prior to this period, the fats consumed by most people came from natural sources like butter, lard, and olive oil. These fats were not only integral to traditional diets but also provided essential nutrients and supported overall health. However, with the advent of industrialization, the food industry sought ways to increase efficiency and profitability. Enter the era of seed and vegetable oils, products derived from crops such as soybeans, corn, cottonseed, and canola.

These oils were initially by-products of other industrial processes and found a new market as cheap alternatives to traditional fats. The marketing campaigns of the time capitalized on emerging scientific studies that linked saturated fats with heart disease, promoting vegetable oils as the heart-healthy choice. The American Heart Association and other influential health organizations endorsed these oils, setting the stage for their widespread acceptance and consumption.

However, beneath the surface of these endorsements and marketing campaigns lay a darker truth. The process of extracting oil from seeds often involves high heat and chemical solvents, which can result in the production of harmful compounds. Furthermore, these oils are high in polyunsaturated fats, which are prone to oxidation—a process that generates free radicals and contributes to inflammation and cellular damage. The shift from traditional fats to seed and vegetable oils marked a significant change in the human diet, one that our bodies have not adapted to over the relatively short span of a few generations.

The hidden crisis in our food is multifaceted. On one hand, it involves the biochemical implications of consuming these oils. On the other, it encompasses the socio-economic and political factors that have driven their adoption. The influence of powerful agricultural and industrial lobbies has shaped dietary guidelines and public health policies, often at the expense of scientific integrity and public well-being. This has led to a situation where many people, including healthcare professionals, are unaware of the true impact of these oils on health.

One of the most insidious aspects of this crisis is its pervasiveness. Seed and vegetable oils are ubiquitous in the modern diet, found in everything from salad dressings and snack foods to baked goods and restaurant meals. Their presence is so widespread that avoiding them requires a concerted and informed effort—something that is beyond the reach of many due to lack of knowledge or resources. This ubiquitous presence contributes to the silent accumulation of health issues over time, manifesting as chronic conditions like heart disease, obesity, diabetes, and inflammatory disorders.

The biochemical effects of these oils are profound. Polyunsaturated fats, while essential in small amounts, can disrupt cellular functions when consumed in excess. These fats are incorporated into cell membranes, affecting their fluidity and function. Moreover, the oxidation of these fats generates reactive oxygen species (ROS), which can damage cellular components, including DNA, proteins, and lipids. This oxidative stress is a key driver of chronic inflammation, a common denominator in many chronic diseases.

Compounding this biochemical assault is the way these oils affect metabolism. Seed and vegetable oils can interfere with insulin signaling, leading to insulin resistance—a precursor to type 2 diabetes. They also contribute to the imbalance of omega-6 and omega-3 fatty acids in the diet, further promoting inflammation. The high caloric density of these oils can lead to weight gain and obesity, creating a vicious cycle of metabolic dysfunction.

Beyond the biochemical and physiological effects, the hidden crisis in our food has significant socio-economic dimensions. The promotion of seed and vegetable oils has been driven by powerful agribusinesses and supported by governmental policies that favor large-scale monoculture farming. These policies have economic ramifications, contributing to the decline of small farms and the erosion of local food systems. The reliance on monoculture crops also has environmental consequences, including soil degradation, loss of biodiversity, and increased pesticide use.

Moreover, the financial entanglements between industry and academia have compromised the integrity of scientific research. Studies funded by the food industry often produce results that favor their sponsors, leading to biased conclusions and recommendations. This has created a landscape where public health policies and dietary guidelines are not always aligned with the best available science. The result is a population that is misinformed about the true impact of their dietary choices.

Addressing the hidden crisis in our food requires a multifaceted approach. Public awareness is a critical first step. People need to be informed about the sources and effects of seed and vegetable oils, and how to recognize and avoid them. This can be achieved through education campaigns, updated dietary guidelines, and clearer food labeling. Healthcare professionals also need to be educated about the latest research on dietary fats and their impact on health, enabling them to provide better guidance to their patients.

At the policy level, there needs to be a reevaluation of agricultural subsidies and support for sustainable farming practices. Encouraging the production and consumption of traditional, nutrient-dense fats can help restore the balance in our diets. Research funding should be directed towards independent studies that explore the long-term effects of dietary fats on health, free from industry influence.

Ultimately, the hidden crisis in our food is a complex interplay of science, economics, and politics. It is a crisis that affects not only our physical health but also the health of our communities and our planet. By uncovering the truth about seed and vegetable oils and advocating for healthier alternatives, we can begin to heal the damage and pave the way for a future where food truly nourishes and sustains us. This journey of healing starts with awareness and is propelled by informed action—both at the individual and collective levels.

Understanding Dark Calories

In the realm of nutrition and wellness, the concept of "dark calories" has emerged as a critical factor in understanding the hidden forces behind many modern health problems. Dark calories are calories derived from foods and substances that contribute to various health issues despite their seemingly benign appearance. These are not just empty calories, which provide no nutritional value; dark calories actively undermine health by promoting inflammation, oxidative stress, and metabolic dysfunction. A primary source of dark calories in the modern diet is seed and vegetable oils.

Seed oils, including those derived from soybeans, corn, cottonseed, and canola, have become staples in many processed foods and cooking practices. Their rise to prominence is a result of industrial processes that enable their mass production at low cost. However, these oils are not as healthful as once believed. To understand dark calories, we need to delve into the biochemistry of these oils, their metabolic effects, and the broader implications of their consumption.

The Biochemistry of Seed Oils

Seed and vegetable oils are high in polyunsaturated fatty acids (PUFAs), particularly omega-6 fatty acids. While our bodies need small amounts of omega-6 fatty acids for normal functioning, the modern diet often contains an excessive amount of these fats, leading to an imbalance between omega-6 and omega-3 fatty acids. This imbalance is a key driver of inflammation in the body.

The process of extracting these oils from seeds typically involves high heat and chemical solvents, which can damage the delicate fatty acids and lead to the formation of harmful compounds such as trans fats and lipid peroxides. These compounds are not only pro-inflammatory but also cytotoxic, meaning they can damage cells directly. When consumed, they integrate into cell membranes, affecting their fluidity and function, and contribute to the creation of advanced glycation end products (AGEs) and reactive oxygen species (ROS). These substances further drive oxidative stress and inflammation.

Metabolic Dysfunction and Dark Calories

The high intake of omega-6 PUFAs from seed and vegetable oils can disrupt several metabolic pathways. One significant impact is on insulin signaling. Omega-6 fats can interfere with the function of insulin receptors on cell surfaces, promoting insulin resistance. This condition is a precursor to type 2 diabetes and is closely linked with obesity, another common issue exacerbated by dark calories.

Additionally, omega-6 fatty acids are prone to oxidation, which means they easily form free radicals—unstable molecules that damage cells, proteins, and DNA. This oxidative stress is a major factor in the development of chronic diseases such as cardiovascular disease, cancer, and neurodegenerative conditions. For example, oxidized LDL cholesterol (a type of cholesterol carrying lipid peroxides) is more likely to contribute to the formation of arterial plaques, leading to heart disease.

Another pathway through which dark calories exert their effects is through the disruption of mitochondrial function. Mitochondria, the powerhouses of the cell, are responsible for producing energy. However, the presence of oxidized fats and other harmful compounds can impair mitochondrial function, leading to decreased energy production and increased production of ROS. This creates a feedback loop of damage and dysfunction.

Dark Calories and Inflammation

Chronic inflammation is a hallmark of many modern diseases, and dark calories play a pivotal role in its perpetuation. When omega-6 fatty acids are metabolized, they give rise to eicosanoids—molecules that can either promote or resolve inflammation. The eicosanoids derived from omega-6 fatty acids, such as prostaglandins and leukotrienes, tend to be pro-inflammatory, promoting the inflammatory response.

The chronic, low-grade inflammation driven by these eicosanoids is subtle and often goes unnoticed until it manifests as a full-blown disease. This type of inflammation contributes to the progression of conditions like arthritis, inflammatory bowel disease, and even depression. In fact, there is growing evidence that inflammation in the body can influence brain function, potentially leading to mood disorders and cognitive decline.

The Impact on Mental Health

The brain is highly susceptible to oxidative stress and inflammation due to its high oxygen consumption and lipid content. Dark calories, particularly those from oxidized fats, can cross the blood-brain barrier and contribute to neuroinflammation. This process can disrupt neurotransmitter balance, impair synaptic function, and damage neurons. The result is an increased risk of mental health issues such as depression, anxiety, and cognitive impairments.

Moreover, dark calories can influence brain energy metabolism. The brain relies heavily on glucose and, to a lesser extent, ketones for energy. However, oxidative stress can impair glucose metabolism, leading to energy deficits in the brain. This energy disruption can affect mood, concentration, and overall mental performance.

The Broader Implications

The implications of consuming dark calories extend beyond individual health to societal and environmental levels. The industrial production of seed oils involves large-scale monoculture farming, which has significant environmental impacts. These farming practices deplete soil nutrients, reduce biodiversity, and increase reliance on chemical fertilizers and pesticides. The environmental degradation associated with these practices contributes to broader ecological imbalances and poses long-term sustainability challenges.

Societally, the promotion and consumption of seed oils are intertwined with economic interests and regulatory policies. The powerful influence of agribusiness and food industry lobbying has shaped dietary guidelines and public health policies in ways that often prioritize profit over public well-being. This has led to a situation where unhealthy food choices are not only prevalent but also often cheaper and more accessible than healthier alternatives.

The financial and healthcare burden of diseases linked to dark calories is enormous. Chronic diseases driven by poor diet and lifestyle choices account for a significant portion of healthcare costs and are leading causes of mortality worldwide. Addressing the root causes of these diseases requires a paradigm shift in how we view food and nutrition.

Moving Forward: Solutions and Strategies

Understanding dark calories is the first step towards mitigating their impact. This knowledge empowers individuals to make informed dietary choices and advocate for healthier food environments. Here are some strategies to reduce the intake of dark calories and promote overall health:

Eliminate or Reduce Seed Oils: Replace seed and vegetable oils with healthier fats such as olive oil, coconut oil, avocado oil, and butter. These fats are less prone to oxidation and provide beneficial nutrients.

Increase Omega-3 Intake: Consume more foods rich in omega-3 fatty acids, such as fatty fish, flaxseeds, and walnuts, to balance the ratio of omega-6 to omega-3 in your diet. Omega-3s have anti-inflammatory properties and support overall health.

Choose Whole, Unprocessed Foods: Focus on whole, minimally processed foods that are naturally nutrient-dense. This includes fresh vegetables, fruits, whole grains, nuts, seeds, and lean proteins.

Read Labels Carefully: Be vigilant about reading ingredient labels to identify and avoid hidden sources of seed and vegetable oils. This includes checking for terms like soybean oil, corn oil, and canola oil.

Support Sustainable Farming Practices: Whenever possible, choose products from sources that prioritize sustainable and regenerative farming practices. This not only supports your health but also the health of the planet.

Advocate for Policy Change: Support initiatives and policies that promote transparency in food labeling, reduce subsidies for harmful agricultural practices, and encourage research into the health effects of different dietary fats.

Educate Yourself and Others: Stay informed about the latest research on nutrition and health, and share this knowledge with others. Building a community of informed consumers can drive demand for healthier food options.

Dark calories represent a hidden threat in our food system, undermining health through their pervasive presence and insidious effects. By understanding the biochemistry and metabolic consequences of seed and vegetable oils, we can make informed choices that support our health and well-being. This understanding also highlights the need for broader changes in our food system, from individual dietary habits to agricultural practices and public health policies. By addressing the issue of dark calories, we take a crucial step towards a healthier future for ourselves and the planet.

PART I: THE DARK SIDE OF SEED OILS AND VEGETABLE OILS

This part delves into the hidden dangers lurking in our food supply, focusing on the rise and proliferation of seed and vegetable oils. It begins with a historical perspective, tracing the transformation of these oils from industrial byproducts to dietary staples. The chapters in this part expose the influence of big industry, unmask the concept of "dark calories," and explain how these harmful oils affect our bodies on a biochemical level. By the end of this section, you will have a deep understanding of the health impacts of seed and vegetable oils, including their role in chronic inflammation, oxidative stress, metabolic disorders, and mental health issues.

1) THE RISE OF VEGETABLE OILS

Historical Background: Vegetable oils have a long and complex history. This chapter traces their rise from industrial byproducts to dietary staples, examining how economic and political forces shaped their prevalence in our diets. Understanding this history is key to understanding why these oils are so deeply embedded in our food culture.

The Influence of Big Industry: The food industry has played a significant role in promoting vegetable oils as healthy alternatives. This section explores how big industry interests have influenced scientific research, public policy, and consumer perceptions to ensure the widespread adoption of these oils, often at the expense of public health.

Evolution of Dietary Guidelines: Dietary guidelines have evolved over the decades, often reflecting industry influence rather than scientific consensus. This chapter examines how guidelines promoting vegetable oils came to be, highlighting the disconnect between official recommendations and emerging scientific evidence about their harmful effects.

Historical Background

The journey of vegetable oils from obscure by-products to ubiquitous staples in modern diets is a fascinating story of industrial innovation, marketing prowess, and scientific influence. This transformation, which took place over the last century, has profoundly shaped dietary habits and health outcomes worldwide. To understand how vegetable oils came to dominate our kitchens and food products, we must delve into their historical background, exploring the socio-economic and scientific forces that propelled their rise.

Historically, the fats and oils consumed by humans were primarily derived from animal sources, such as lard, tallow, and butter, as well as from plant sources like olives, coconuts, and avocados. These fats were integral to traditional diets across various cultures, valued not only for their flavor and cooking properties but also for their essential nutrients. For example, olive oil, prized in Mediterranean cuisine, was revered for its health benefits and rich flavor, while coconut oil was a staple in tropical regions.

In many traditional diets, these fats provided a balanced intake of essential fatty acids, vitamins, and energy. The dietary patterns of indigenous populations and rural communities often featured a variety of fats, tailored to local agriculture and environment. These fats were consumed in their whole, unprocessed forms, maintaining their nutritional integrity and health benefits.

The shift from traditional fats to vegetable oils began with the Industrial Revolution in the 19th century. This period was marked by significant advancements in technology and manufacturing, which laid the groundwork for the large-scale production of vegetable oils. The development of steam-powered machinery and the chemical solvents necessary for oil extraction made it possible to process seeds and grains on an industrial scale.

In the early 1900s, the demand for cheap and stable fats grew, driven by the needs of an expanding urban population and the food industry's quest for efficiency and cost reduction. At this time, cottonseed oil emerged as one of the first major vegetable oils to be processed on a large scale. Cottonseed oil was initially a by-product of the cotton industry, and its utilization helped reduce waste and create a new revenue stream. Its production was further bolstered by the development of the hydraulic press, which made oil extraction more efficient.

A pivotal moment in the history of vegetable oils was the discovery of their potential health benefits, particularly in relation to cholesterol and heart disease. In the 20th century, scientific research began to explore the links between dietary fats and cardiovascular health. An important figure in this narrative was Ancel Keys, an American physiologist whose research in the 1950s suggested a connection between saturated fats and heart disease. Keys' studies led to the development of the "lipid hypothesis," which posited that saturated fats raised blood cholesterol levels and increased the risk of heart disease.

This hypothesis gained widespread acceptance, and public health campaigns began to promote the consumption of polyunsaturated fats, such as those found in vegetable oils, as a healthier alternative to saturated fats. The idea was that substituting saturated fats with polyunsaturated fats would lower cholesterol levels and reduce the risk of heart disease. This theory was further bolstered by the introduction of hydrogenation, a process that made liquid oils more solid and stable, extending their shelf life and enhancing their utility in food products.

The endorsement of vegetable oils by the scientific community and health organizations set the stage for a massive marketing campaign that would shape consumer preferences for decades. Companies invested heavily in advertising, promoting vegetable oils as modern, healthful alternatives to traditional fats. Campaigns highlighted the supposed health benefits of these oils, emphasizing their ability to lower cholesterol and prevent heart disease.

This marketing push was supported by legislative and regulatory changes. In the United States, the 1960s saw the introduction of food labeling regulations that encouraged the use of vegetable oils in processed foods. The Food and Drug Administration (FDA) and other regulatory bodies began to endorse the use of polyunsaturated fats, further legitimizing their place in the diet. The American Heart Association (AHA), a powerful advocate for heart health, endorsed vegetable oils, reinforcing their image as a heart-healthy choice.

During this time, the production of soybean oil skyrocketed, driven by agricultural subsidies and research grants that supported its cultivation. The soybean industry, in particular, flourished, becoming one of the largest producers of vegetable oils. The proliferation of soybean oil, alongside other seed oils like corn, sunflower, and canola, became a defining feature of the modern food supply.

As the health benefits of vegetable oils became widely accepted, the food industry embraced them wholeheartedly. The transition from traditional fats to vegetable oils was swift and extensive, transforming the composition of countless food products. Margarine, once considered an inferior substitute for butter, became a popular choice, marketed as a healthier option with its low saturated fat content. Snack foods, baked goods, and fast foods increasingly featured vegetable oils, leveraging their stability, flavor, and ability to enhance texture and shelf life.

The shift was not without controversy. Some critics argued that the promotion of vegetable oils was driven more by economic interests than by sound science. The influence of agribusiness and food manufacturers on scientific research and public policy became a focal point of debate. Critics pointed out that the studies supporting the health benefits of vegetable oils were often funded by the industries that stood to gain from their promotion. This conflict of interest raised questions about the integrity of the research and the validity of the guidelines that recommended these oils.

As the consumption of vegetable oils increased, so did the incidence of chronic diseases. The health benefits touted by early proponents of these oils began to be questioned as epidemiological studies and clinical trials failed to confirm the expected reductions in heart disease. In fact, the rising rates of obesity, diabetes, and inflammatory conditions suggested that something was amiss.

Research began to uncover the darker side of vegetable oils. The high content of omega-6 polyunsaturated fats, while essential in small amounts, was shown to promote inflammation when consumed in excess. The process of refining and hydrogenating these oils created trans fats and oxidized lipids, both of which are harmful to health. The imbalance between omega-6 and omega-3 fatty acids, exacerbated by the dominance of vegetable oils in the diet, was linked to a host of chronic conditions, from cardiovascular disease to neurodegenerative disorders.

In recent years, there has been a growing recognition of the need to revisit dietary recommendations regarding fats. Scientists, nutritionists, and health advocates are increasingly calling for a reevaluation of the role of vegetable oils in the diet. The focus is shifting towards whole, minimally processed fats, such as olive oil, coconut oil, and animal fats, which have been shown to support health in ways that vegetable oils cannot.

This shift is supported by a growing body of evidence suggesting that the benefits of traditional fats, such as those found in Mediterranean diets, are real and significant. These fats are rich in monounsaturated fats and omega-3 fatty acids, which have anti-inflammatory properties and support overall health. As the public becomes more informed, there is a growing demand for transparency in food labeling and a return to more traditional, nutrient-dense foods.

The rise of vegetable oils is a story of innovation, marketing, and the evolution of dietary norms. From their origins as industrial by-products to their current status as dietary staples, vegetable oils have undergone a remarkable transformation. This journey, however, has not been without its challenges and consequences. The shift towards vegetable oils, driven by scientific assumptions and economic interests, has had profound implications for public health. As we continue to uncover the complexities of nutrition and health, the lessons from this history remind us of the importance of critical thinking, scientific integrity, and a balanced approach to diet and wellness. The journey forward involves re-evaluating our choices and embracing foods that truly nourish and support our health.

The Influence of Big Industry

The ascent of vegetable oils to a dominant position in the global food market is not solely the result of scientific discovery and health advocacy; it has also been significantly shaped by the powerful influence of big industry. From agricultural giants to multinational food corporations, various sectors have played a critical role in promoting and entrenching vegetable oils in our diets. This influence has been exerted through strategic investments, marketing campaigns, and lobbying efforts that have reshaped public perceptions and dietary guidelines.

In the early 20th century, the burgeoning industrial sector recognized the economic potential of vegetable oils. Initially, these oils were by-products of other agricultural processes, such as cotton production, and their utilization represented an opportunity to reduce waste and generate additional revenue. This pragmatic approach quickly evolved into a full-fledged industry as technological advancements made it possible to extract oil from a variety of seeds, including soybeans, corn, and sunflowers.

The development of the hydrogenation process in the early 1900s was a game-changer for the vegetable oil industry. Hydrogenation, which converts liquid oils into solid or semi-solid fats, extended the shelf life of oils and created versatile products like margarine. Companies like Procter & Gamble capitalized on this innovation, marketing Crisco, a hydrogenated cottonseed oil product, as a superior alternative to traditional cooking fats. This marked the beginning of a concerted effort by industry players to promote vegetable oils as modern and healthy choices.

Marketing played a pivotal role in shaping consumer preferences. Throughout the mid-20th century, food companies launched extensive advertising campaigns to persuade the public of the benefits of vegetable oils. These campaigns often featured endorsements from scientists and health professionals, lending credibility to the claims. The narrative that vegetable oils were healthier than animal fats became deeply ingrained in the public consciousness, largely due to these well-funded marketing efforts.

In addition to marketing, the food industry exerted influence through strategic partnerships and lobbying. Major food corporations collaborated with scientific researchers and health organizations to promote the lipid hypothesis—the theory that dietary saturated fats raise cholesterol levels and increase the risk of heart disease. The American Heart Association (AHA), among other influential bodies, endorsed this hypothesis and recommended the substitution of saturated fats with polyunsaturated fats from vegetable oils.

These endorsements were not without controversy. Critics argued that the research supporting the lipid hypothesis was often funded by the very industries that stood to benefit from the promotion of vegetable oils. This conflict of interest raised questions about the objectivity of the scientific findings and the validity of the dietary recommendations. Nonetheless, the combined efforts of industry, science, and public health organizations successfully shifted dietary guidelines towards increased consumption of vegetable oils.

Government policies also played a crucial role in promoting vegetable oils. Agricultural subsidies in the United States, for example, favored the production of oilseed crops like soybeans and corn. These subsidies made these crops economically attractive to farmers and ensured a steady supply of raw materials for the vegetable oil industry. The alignment of agricultural policy with industrial interests created a powerful synergy that further entrenched vegetable oils in the food supply.

The influence of big industry extended to global markets as well. Multinational corporations expanded their reach, promoting vegetable oils in developing countries through trade agreements and marketing initiatives. These efforts were often supported by international development agencies that viewed the adoption of vegetable oils as a means to address food security and malnutrition. As a result, vegetable oils became staples in diets worldwide, contributing to a shift away from traditional fats in many cultures.

The food industry's influence on dietary habits has had significant health implications. The widespread adoption of vegetable oils has coincided with rising rates of chronic diseases, such as obesity, diabetes, and cardiovascular disease. While early proponents of vegetable oils touted their benefits, subsequent research has revealed potential downsides. The high levels of omega-6 fatty acids in many vegetable oils, for instance, have been linked to inflammation and various health issues.

Despite these concerns, the vegetable oil industry continues to wield considerable influence. Food manufacturers rely on these oils for their versatility and cost-effectiveness, and they remain a staple in processed foods, fast foods, and restaurant cooking. The industry's ability to adapt to changing market conditions and consumer preferences ensures that vegetable oils remain a prominent feature of the modern diet.

In recent years, there has been a growing movement to challenge the dominance of vegetable oils and promote healthier alternatives. Advocates for traditional fats, such as olive oil, coconut oil, and butter, emphasize the nutritional benefits of these whole, minimally processed fats. This shift is supported by emerging research that highlights the importance of a balanced intake of fatty acids and the potential harms of an over-reliance on omega-6-rich vegetable oils.

The influence of big industry on the rise of vegetable oils is a testament to the power of economic and strategic interests in shaping dietary patterns. The coordinated efforts of agricultural producers, food manufacturers, marketers, and policymakers have transformed vegetable oils from industrial by-products into dietary staples. As we continue to explore the complex relationship between diet and health, it is crucial to remain mindful of the forces that drive our food choices and to advocate for transparency, integrity, and balance in nutritional guidance. The journey towards healthier eating requires a critical examination of past influences and a commitment to informed, evidence-based decisions for the future.

Evolution of Dietary Guidelines

The evolution of dietary guidelines, particularly regarding the consumption of fats and oils, has been significantly influenced by scientific research, public health initiatives, and the powerful food industry. These guidelines have undergone substantial changes over the past century, reflecting shifts in scientific understanding, health priorities, and economic interests. Understanding this evolution is crucial to comprehending how vegetable oils came to dominate our diets and the broader implications for public health.

In the early 20th century, dietary guidelines were relatively simple and focused on preventing nutrient deficiencies. The primary concern was ensuring adequate intake of essential nutrients like vitamins, minerals, and proteins. Fats, including butter, lard, and other animal fats, were considered valuable sources of energy and essential fatty acids. Traditional fats were an integral part of the diet, and there was little differentiation between types of fats regarding health impacts.

The shift towards emphasizing the types of fats in the diet began in the mid-20th century with the emergence of the lipid hypothesis. This theory, popularized by researchers such as Ancel Keys, posited that dietary saturated fats raised blood cholesterol levels, which in turn increased the risk of heart disease. Keys' Seven Countries Study, published in the 1950s, played a pivotal role in linking saturated fat consumption with coronary heart disease, although later critiques highlighted methodological flaws and selective data use.

The lipid hypothesis gained significant traction and led to a major paradigm shift in dietary guidelines. By the 1960s and 1970s, public health organizations, including the American Heart Association (AHA) and government bodies, began advocating for reduced intake of saturated fats and cholesterol. The focus was on promoting polyunsaturated fats, particularly those found in vegetable oils, as healthier alternatives. This shift was based on the belief that replacing saturated fats with polyunsaturated fats would lower cholesterol levels and reduce heart disease risk.

These recommendations were codified in the 1977 Dietary Goals for the United States, a report issued by the U.S. Senate Select Committee on Nutrition and Human Needs. The report recommended that Americans reduce their intake of total fat, saturated fat, and cholesterol while increasing their consumption of carbohydrates and polyunsaturated fats. This marked the beginning of a low-fat, high-carbohydrate dietary era that would dominate nutritional guidelines for decades.

The food industry quickly adapted to these new guidelines, reformulating products to reduce saturated fat content and increase the use of vegetable oils. Margarine, once promoted as a healthier alternative to butter, became a staple in American households. Processed foods were marketed with "low-fat" and "cholesterol-free" labels, capitalizing on the growing public concern about heart disease and the perceived benefits of vegetable oils.

However, the low-fat, high-carbohydrate dietary recommendations did not lead to the expected decline in heart disease rates. Instead, obesity and related metabolic disorders, such as type 2 diabetes, began to rise dramatically. This paradox prompted researchers to re-examine the scientific basis of the dietary guidelines and explore the potential unintended consequences of promoting low-fat diets.

In the 1980s and 1990s, new research started to challenge the lipid hypothesis and the blanket recommendation to reduce all fats. Studies began to differentiate between types of fats, highlighting the health benefits of monounsaturated and certain polyunsaturated fats, such as omega-3 fatty acids. The Mediterranean diet, rich in olive oil, fish, nuts, and whole foods, gained attention for its association with lower rates of heart disease and overall mortality, despite its relatively high-fat content.

The 2000s saw further revisions to dietary guidelines as the understanding of fats became more nuanced. The 2005 Dietary Guidelines for Americans acknowledged the health benefits of unsaturated fats and recommended replacing saturated fats with monounsaturated and polyunsaturated fats rather than simply reducing total fat intake. This shift reflected a growing recognition that the type of fat consumed is more important than the total amount.

In 2015, the Dietary Guidelines for Americans took a significant step by removing the longstanding recommendation to limit dietary cholesterol. This change was based on accumulating evidence that dietary cholesterol has a relatively small impact on blood cholesterol levels for most people. The guidelines continued to emphasize the importance of healthy fats while advising limits on saturated fat intake.

Despite these advancements, the influence of the food industry on dietary guidelines remains a contentious issue. Critics argue that industry interests have at times shaped nutritional recommendations to favor processed foods and vegetable oils. The role of industry-funded research in supporting favorable guidelines and the impact of lobbying efforts on policy decisions have raised concerns about the integrity of public health recommendations.

Moreover, the guidelines' emphasis on reducing saturated fats has been criticized for potentially leading to increased consumption of refined carbohydrates and sugars, which have their own adverse health effects. The unintended consequence of promoting low-fat products often resulted in foods with higher sugar content, contributing to the obesity and diabetes epidemics.

As of the early 2020s, dietary guidelines continue to evolve in response to new research and changing public health priorities. There is a growing emphasis on whole foods, dietary patterns, and the overall quality of the diet rather than focusing on individual nutrients. The recognition of the importance of dietary fats in maintaining health has led to more balanced recommendations that encourage the consumption of healthy fats from sources like olive oil, nuts, seeds, and fatty fish.

The evolution of dietary guidelines reflects the dynamic nature of nutritional science and the complex interplay between research, industry, and public policy. While the promotion of vegetable oils was initially based on the best available evidence and public health goals, subsequent developments have highlighted the need for a more holistic and balanced approach to dietary recommendations. Understanding this history helps us appreciate the challenges and opportunities in crafting guidelines that truly promote health and well-being.

The future of dietary guidelines will likely continue to integrate emerging scientific insights with a focus on whole, minimally processed foods. There is a growing movement towards personalized nutrition, recognizing that individual health responses to dietary components can vary widely. As we move forward, the lessons learned from the rise of vegetable oils and the evolution of dietary guidelines underscore the importance of scientific rigor, transparency, and adaptability in promoting public health.

2) UNMASKING DARK CALORIES

Defining Dark Calories: Dark calories are the hidden, harmful energy sources in our diets, primarily from seed and vegetable oils. This section provides a detailed definition of dark calories, explaining how they differ from regular calories and why they are particularly damaging to our health.

The Biochemistry of Harmful Oils: This chapter delves into the biochemical mechanisms by which seed and vegetable oils cause harm. It explains how these oils interact with our cells, leading to inflammation, oxidative stress, and other negative health outcomes. Understanding this science is crucial for grasping the full impact of these oils on our bodies.

How Dark Calories Affect Our Bodies: Dark calories have a wide range of effects on our health, from metabolic disorders to mental health issues. This section explores these effects in detail, providing a comprehensive overview of how harmful oils disrupt various bodily systems and contribute to chronic disease.

Defining Dark Calories

The term "dark calories" refers to a hidden and insidious element in our diet that contributes to numerous health issues without providing substantial nutritional benefits. Unlike empty calories, which simply offer little nutritional value, dark calories actively promote adverse health effects. Understanding and defining dark calories is crucial for anyone seeking to improve their diet and overall health. These calories are primarily associated with highly processed and refined foods, particularly those high in certain vegetable and seed oils that have undergone significant industrial processing.

Dark calories are largely derived from oils such as soybean oil, corn oil, sunflower oil, and other commonly used vegetable oils. These oils are heavily processed and chemically altered to enhance their shelf life and cooking properties, but in the process, they lose much of their natural nutrient profile and gain harmful properties. The refining process often involves high heat and the use of solvents, which can strip away beneficial compounds and introduce harmful substances.

The concept of dark calories extends beyond the simple notion of calories being a measure of energy. It encompasses the quality and source of those calories, emphasizing that not all calories are created equal. Calories from dark sources not only fail to provide essential nutrients but also carry compounds that can disrupt metabolic processes and promote chronic inflammation, oxidative stress, and other health issues.

At the heart of dark calories is the imbalance of omega-6 to omega-3 fatty acids. Omega-6 fatty acids, while essential in small amounts, are pro-inflammatory when consumed in excess. The modern diet, dominated by vegetable oils, has dramatically skewed this balance, leading to an overconsumption of omega-6 fatty acids. Historically, humans evolved on a diet with a roughly 1:1 ratio of omega-6 to omega-3 fatty acids. However, contemporary diets can have ratios as high as 20:1 or even 30:1. This imbalance contributes to a host of health problems, including heart disease, diabetes, obesity, and various inflammatory conditions.

The refining process that creates dark calories also produces trans fats and oxidized lipids, both of which are detrimental to health. Trans fats, created through partial hydrogenation, are well-known for their role in increasing bad cholesterol (LDL) and decreasing good cholesterol (HDL), thereby raising the risk of heart disease. Although many countries have taken steps to reduce or ban trans fats, they still linger in some processed foods. Oxidized lipids, on the other hand, form when oils are exposed to heat, light, and oxygen during processing. These oxidized compounds can cause oxidative stress in the body, damaging cells and contributing to chronic diseases such as cancer and neurodegenerative disorders.

Dark calories are also linked to the pervasive presence of processed foods in the modern diet. These foods are often high in refined carbohydrates and sugars in addition to unhealthy oils, creating a potent combination that drives metabolic dysfunction.

Processed foods are designed to be hyper-palatable, exploiting our natural cravings for fat, sugar, and salt, and leading to overconsumption. This overconsumption not only leads to excessive caloric intake but also displaces healthier, nutrient-dense foods from the diet.

The biochemical impact of dark calories extends to the cellular level. Consuming these calories disrupts normal metabolic processes, leading to insulin resistance, impaired glucose metabolism, and increased fat storage, particularly visceral fat, which surrounds internal organs and is associated with higher risks of metabolic syndrome, type 2 diabetes, and cardiovascular diseases. Additionally, the inflammation promoted by an excess of omega-6 fatty acids can exacerbate these conditions, creating a vicious cycle of poor health.

Another crucial aspect of dark calories is their impact on the brain and mental health. The imbalance of fatty acids affects brain function, contributing to cognitive decline, mood disorders, and mental health issues. Studies have shown that diets high in processed vegetable oils are associated with increased rates of depression and anxiety. The inflammatory effects of these oils can alter neurotransmitter function and disrupt the delicate balance of brain chemistry.

One of the most insidious features of dark calories is their ubiquity. Vegetable oils and their derivatives are found in a vast array of processed foods, from snack items and fast foods to seemingly healthy products like salad dressings and granola bars. This pervasive presence makes it challenging for consumers to avoid dark calories without a concerted effort to read labels and make informed choices. The food industry's reliance on these oils is driven by their low cost, long shelf life, and desirable cooking properties, such as high smoke points and neutral flavors, which make them versatile ingredients in processed foods.

The concept of dark calories also encompasses the deceptive marketing tactics used to promote these oils as healthy options. Many vegetable oils are marketed as heart-healthy due to their unsaturated fat content, yet this marketing often overlooks the negative health impacts of excessive omega-6 fatty acids and the harmful effects of processing. The promotion of these oils as cholesterol-lowering agents further complicates the public's understanding of their health implications, as the focus on cholesterol has overshadowed the broader context of overall dietary quality and balance.

To combat the negative health effects of dark calories, it is essential to shift towards a diet that emphasizes whole, unprocessed foods and healthy fats. This includes incorporating oils that are minimally processed and have a balanced fatty acid profile, such as extra virgin olive oil, coconut oil, and avocado oil. These oils not only provide essential nutrients but also have anti-inflammatory properties that support overall health. Additionally, consuming a diet rich in omega-3 fatty acids, found in fatty fish, flaxseeds, and chia seeds, can help restore the balance of fatty acids and mitigate the inflammatory effects of excess omega-6.

Educating consumers about the sources and impacts of dark calories is a crucial step in promoting healthier dietary choices. This includes understanding food labels, recognizing hidden sources of unhealthy oils, and being aware of marketing tactics that can mislead consumers. Public health initiatives and policy changes that promote transparency and prioritize nutritional quality over industrial interests are essential for creating a food environment that supports health rather than undermines it.

In summary, defining dark calories involves recognizing the detrimental impact of highly processed vegetable oils and their widespread presence in the modern diet. These calories contribute to chronic inflammation, metabolic dysfunction, and a range of health issues, all while offering little to no nutritional benefit. Addressing the problem of dark calories requires a comprehensive approach that includes dietary changes, consumer education, and policy reform to promote a healthier, more balanced food environment. By understanding and unmasking dark calories, individuals can take proactive steps towards better health and well-being

The Biochemistry of Harmful Oils

Understanding the biochemistry of harmful oils is key to recognizing how they contribute to the phenomenon of dark calories and the subsequent health issues that arise from their consumption. These oils, primarily derived from seeds such as soybeans, corn, sunflower, and safflower, undergo extensive industrial processing that transforms their biochemical nature, often rendering them detrimental to human health.

Extraction and Refining Process

The initial step in the production of vegetable oils involves extracting the oil from the seeds. This is typically done using mechanical pressing or chemical solvents like hexane. Mechanical pressing, while somewhat less intrusive, does not extract as much oil as solvent extraction. The chemical method involves soaking the seeds in the solvent to dissolve the oil, which is then separated from the solvent through evaporation. Although the solvent is removed, traces can remain in the final product.

After extraction, the crude oil undergoes refining to remove impurities, odors, and colors. This process includes several stages: degumming, neutralization, bleaching, and deodorization. Degumming removes phospholipids and other impurities. Neutralization involves adding an alkali to remove free fatty acids, which can cause the oil to become rancid. Bleaching removes pigments and other color bodies using bleaching clays. Finally, deodorization uses high heat and steam to remove volatile compounds that contribute to odor and taste.

Each of these steps significantly alters the biochemical composition of the oil. The high temperatures and chemical treatments can strip the oil of beneficial nutrients such as tocopherols (vitamin E), phytosterols, and other antioxidants, while also introducing harmful compounds.

Fatty Acid Composition

One of the most critical aspects of harmful oils lies in their fatty acid composition. Vegetable oils are typically high in polyunsaturated fatty acids (PUFAs), particularly omega-6 fatty acids. While these fatty acids are essential for human health in small amounts, the problem arises with their disproportionate consumption.

Historically, human diets maintained a balanced ratio of omega-6 to omega-3 fatty acids, roughly 1:1 to 4:1. However, the modern diet, heavily laden with vegetable oils, has skewed this ratio to as high as 20:1 or even 30:1. This imbalance fosters an environment ripe for chronic inflammation, as omega-6 fatty acids, particularly linoleic acid, are precursors to pro-inflammatory eicosanoids. These signaling molecules play a role in inflammatory and immune responses, and their overproduction is linked to chronic inflammatory diseases such as heart disease, arthritis, and certain cancers.

Conversely, omega-3 fatty acids, found in flaxseeds, walnuts, and fish oils, produce anti-inflammatory eicosanoids. The excessive intake of omega-6 fatty acids relative to omega-3s overwhelms the body's biochemical pathways, tipping the balance towards inflammation and associated chronic conditions.

Hydrogenation and Trans Fats

Another critical biochemical alteration occurs during the hydrogenation process, commonly used to solidify vegetable oils for products like margarine and shortening. Hydrogenation involves adding hydrogen atoms to the carbon-carbon double bonds of unsaturated fats, converting them into saturated fats and thereby extending the oil's shelf life and stability.

Partial hydrogenation, however, results in the formation of trans fats, which are unsaturated fats with at least one double bond in the trans configuration (opposite sides of the carbon chain). Trans fats are notorious for their adverse health effects. They not only raise levels of low-density lipoprotein (LDL) cholesterol but also lower high-density lipoprotein (HDL) cholesterol, increasing the risk of coronary artery disease. Trans fats are also linked to inflammation, insulin resistance, and diabetes.

Despite regulations and bans in many countries, trans fats still persist in some processed foods, particularly in countries with less stringent food safety regulations.

Oxidative Stress and Lipid Peroxidation

The high levels of polyunsaturated fats in vegetable oils make them particularly prone to oxidation, especially when exposed to heat, light, and oxygen during processing, storage, and cooking. Oxidation leads to the formation of lipid peroxides and aldehydes, highly reactive compounds that cause oxidative stress in the body.

Oxidative stress occurs when there is an imbalance between free radicals (reactive oxygen species) and antioxidants in the body. Free radicals can damage cellular components such as lipids, proteins, and DNA, leading to cellular dysfunction and contributing to the development of chronic diseases such as cancer, neurodegenerative disorders, and cardiovascular diseases.

Lipid peroxides, formed from the oxidation of PUFAs, are particularly damaging. They can initiate chain reactions that propagate further lipid oxidation, creating a cascade of oxidative damage. Aldehydes, another byproduct of lipid peroxidation, are toxic to cells and can cross-link proteins and DNA, impairing their function and leading to cell death.

Impact on Mitochondrial Function

Mitochondria, the energy-producing organelles in cells, are particularly vulnerable to damage from harmful oils. The oxidative stress induced by lipid peroxidation can impair mitochondrial function, leading to reduced energy production and increased production of reactive oxygen species. This creates a vicious cycle where mitochondrial dysfunction leads to more oxidative stress, further damaging cellular components.

Compromised mitochondrial function is associated with a range of metabolic disorders, including obesity, type 2 diabetes, and metabolic syndrome. Mitochondria are also involved in regulating apoptosis (programmed cell death), and their dysfunction can contribute to the development of cancer by allowing damaged cells to survive and proliferate.

Inflammatory Pathways

As previously mentioned, the high omega-6 content in harmful vegetable oils promotes the production of pro-inflammatory eicosanoids. This not only contributes to chronic inflammation but also disrupts normal metabolic processes. Chronic inflammation is a common thread in many chronic diseases, including cardiovascular disease, type 2 diabetes, Alzheimer's disease, and certain cancers.

Moreover, the chronic inflammation induced by excessive omega-6 fatty acid consumption can affect the gut microbiota, leading to dysbiosis (an imbalance in the microbial community). Dysbiosis is linked to a range of health issues, including inflammatory bowel disease, obesity, and metabolic syndrome. The gut microbiota plays a crucial role in regulating immune responses, and its disruption can exacerbate systemic inflammation and metabolic dysfunction.

Insulin Resistance and Metabolic Dysfunction

The biochemical impact of harmful oils extends to insulin signaling pathways. The inflammation and oxidative stress induced by these oils can impair insulin receptor function, leading to insulin resistance. Insulin resistance is a hallmark of metabolic syndrome and is closely associated with obesity, type 2 diabetes, and cardiovascular disease.

Additionally, the high caloric density and hyper-palatable nature of processed foods rich in harmful oils contribute to overeating and weight gain. These foods often contain refined carbohydrates and sugars, further exacerbating insulin resistance and metabolic dysfunction. The combination of high-fat, high-sugar diets creates a metabolic environment that promotes fat storage, particularly visceral fat, which is metabolically active and contributes to systemic inflammation.

Conclusion

The biochemistry of harmful oils reveals a complex interplay of factors that contribute to their classification as dark calories. From the initial extraction and refining processes that strip beneficial nutrients and introduce harmful compounds, to the disproportionate omega-6 fatty acid content that promotes chronic inflammation, these oils pose significant health risks.

Understanding these biochemical mechanisms is crucial for making informed dietary choices. Reducing the intake of harmful oils and replacing them with healthier alternatives, such as extra virgin olive oil, coconut oil, and oils rich in omega-3 fatty acids, can help mitigate the adverse health effects. Additionally, focusing on whole, unprocessed foods and maintaining a balanced diet rich in antioxidants can support overall health and reduce the risk of chronic diseases associated with the consumption of dark calories.

How Dark Calories Affect Our Bodies

The concept of dark calories highlights how certain dietary components, particularly those derived from heavily processed vegetable oils, exert profound negative effects on our health. These dark calories, found in many modern foods, affect our bodies in multiple detrimental ways, contributing to a host of chronic diseases and metabolic disorders. To understand how dark calories impact our health, it's essential to delve into their effects on inflammation, metabolic processes, cellular function, mental health, and overall well-being.

Inflammation and Oxidative Stress

One of the primary ways dark calories harm our bodies is through the promotion of chronic inflammation and oxidative stress. The high omega-6 fatty acid content in many vegetable oils, such as soybean, corn, and sunflower oil, leads to an overproduction of pro-inflammatory eicosanoids. These molecules, derived from arachidonic acid, play a crucial role in the body's inflammatory response. When consumed in excess, omega-6 fatty acids tip the balance towards a pro-inflammatory state, fostering chronic inflammation throughout the body.

Chronic inflammation is a key driver of many chronic diseases, including cardiovascular disease, diabetes, arthritis, and certain cancers. It can damage blood vessels, increase blood pressure, and contribute to the formation of atherosclerotic plaques, leading to heart attacks and strokes. Inflammatory processes also interfere with insulin signaling, promoting insulin resistance, a precursor to type 2 diabetes.

Additionally, the oxidative stress induced by dark calories further exacerbates inflammation. Oxidative stress occurs when there's an imbalance between the production of free radicals and the body's ability to neutralize them with antioxidants. Free radicals, highly reactive molecules, can damage cellular components such as lipids, proteins, and DNA, leading to cellular dysfunction and death. The lipid peroxides and aldehydes formed from the oxidation of polyunsaturated fats in vegetable oils are particularly harmful, perpetuating a cycle of oxidative damage and inflammation.

Metabolic Dysfunction and Obesity

Dark calories also contribute significantly to metabolic dysfunction and obesity. The consumption of heavily processed vegetable oils and the foods containing them often leads to an excess intake of calories without corresponding nutritional benefits. These oils are high in calories but low in essential nutrients, leading to a phenomenon where individuals consume more calories to meet their nutritional needs, promoting weight gain and obesity.

Obesity itself is a major risk factor for numerous health conditions, including type 2 diabetes, cardiovascular disease, and certain cancers. It is characterized by an excess accumulation of body fat, particularly visceral fat, which surrounds internal organs. Visceral fat is metabolically active and releases pro-inflammatory cytokines, further promoting systemic inflammation and metabolic dysfunction.

Moreover, dark calories disrupt normal metabolic processes by impairing insulin signaling. Insulin resistance, where cells become less responsive to insulin, is a hallmark of metabolic syndrome and type 2 diabetes. This condition leads to elevated blood glucose levels, increased fat storage, and a higher risk of cardiovascular disease. The inflammatory and oxidative stress induced by dark calories aggravates insulin resistance, creating a vicious cycle of metabolic dysfunction.

Cellular Damage and Aging

At the cellular level, the impact of dark calories is profound. The oxidative stress and inflammation promoted by these calories accelerate cellular aging and damage. Mitochondria, the energy-producing organelles in cells, are particularly vulnerable. Mitochondrial dysfunction, caused by oxidative damage, leads to reduced energy production, increased production of reactive oxygen species, and impaired cellular function.

This mitochondrial dysfunction is implicated in a range of age-related diseases, including neurodegenerative disorders like Alzheimer's disease, Parkinson's disease, and cardiovascular diseases. The cumulative effect of oxidative damage to DNA, proteins, and lipids over time contributes to the aging process and the development of chronic diseases associated with aging.

Furthermore, dark calories can interfere with normal cellular processes such as apoptosis (programmed cell death) and autophagy (cellular cleanup). Proper regulation of these processes is essential for maintaining cellular health and function. Dysregulation can lead to the survival of damaged cells, increasing the risk of cancer, and impaired autophagy can contribute to the accumulation of cellular debris and dysfunctional proteins, exacerbating neurodegenerative conditions.

Mental Health and Cognitive Function

The impact of dark calories extends to mental health and cognitive function. The brain is highly sensitive to changes in diet and nutrition, and the inflammatory and oxidative stress effects of dark calories can have significant implications for brain health. Diets high in processed vegetable oils are associated with an increased risk of depression, anxiety, and cognitive decline.

The imbalance of omega-6 to omega-3 fatty acids plays a critical role in brain function. Omega-3 fatty acids, particularly docosahexaenoic acid (DHA), are essential for maintaining the structure and function of brain cells. They have anti-inflammatory properties and support neuronal health. A diet high in omega-6 fatty acids, however, can displace omega-3 fatty acids in cell membranes, impairing brain function and increasing the risk of neuroinflammation and cognitive decline.

Inflammation in the brain, driven by an excess of pro-inflammatory eicosanoids, can disrupt neurotransmitter function and brain signaling pathways. This disruption is linked to mood disorders such as depression and anxiety. Additionally, oxidative stress can damage neurons and support cells in the brain, leading to neurodegeneration and impaired cognitive function.

Digestive Health and the Gut Microbiome

Dark calories also negatively affect digestive health and the gut microbiome. The gut microbiome, a complex community of microorganisms living in the digestive tract, plays a crucial role in overall health. It helps with digestion, supports the immune system, and influences metabolic and inflammatory processes.

Dietary intake of harmful oils can disrupt the balance of the gut microbiome, leading to dysbiosis. Dysbiosis is associated with a range of health issues, including inflammatory bowel disease, irritable bowel syndrome, obesity, and metabolic syndrome. The pro-inflammatory effects of dark calories can also contribute to gut inflammation, increasing the risk of conditions like leaky gut syndrome, where the intestinal barrier becomes permeable, allowing toxins and bacteria to enter the bloodstream.

Furthermore, the high calorie, low-nutrient nature of processed foods rich in dark calories can alter gut microbiota composition, favoring the growth of harmful bacteria over beneficial ones. This imbalance can impair nutrient absorption, further exacerbating nutritional deficiencies and promoting systemic inflammation.

Cardiovascular Health

Cardiovascular health is profoundly impacted by the consumption of dark calories. The inflammation and oxidative stress promoted by these calories can damage blood vessels, leading to the development of atherosclerosis (hardening of the arteries). Atherosclerosis is characterized by the buildup of plaques in the arterial walls, which can restrict blood flow and lead to heart attacks, strokes, and other cardiovascular events.

The high intake of omega-6 fatty acids and trans fats from partially hydrogenated oils raises LDL cholesterol levels and lowers HDL cholesterol levels, increasing the risk of coronary artery disease. Trans fats, in particular, have been shown to increase the risk of heart disease significantly, prompting many health organizations to recommend their elimination from the diet.

In addition, the pro-inflammatory state induced by dark calories contributes to hypertension (high blood pressure), a major risk factor for cardiovascular disease. Inflammation can cause blood vessels to narrow and stiffen, increasing blood pressure and the strain on the heart.

Endocrine Disruption

The chemicals used in the processing of vegetable oils, such as solvents and bleaching agents, can introduce endocrine disruptors into the final product. Endocrine disruptors are chemicals that can interfere with hormone function, leading to a range of health issues. These chemicals can mimic or block hormones, disrupting the body's normal hormonal balance and contributing to conditions such as obesity, diabetes, reproductive disorders, and certain cancers.

Exposure to endocrine disruptors can affect the development and function of the reproductive system, thyroid, and other endocrine glands. For instance, certain compounds used in the refining process of oils can act as estrogen mimics, disrupting the normal balance of sex hormones and potentially increasing the risk of hormone-related cancers such as breast and prostate cancer.

The pervasive impact of dark calories on our bodies underscores the importance of understanding and mitigating their consumption. From promoting chronic inflammation and oxidative stress to disrupting metabolic processes, cellular function, mental health, digestive health, cardiovascular health, and endocrine function, the biochemical effects of dark calories are far-reaching and detrimental.

Reducing the intake of dark calories requires a concerted effort to choose whole, unprocessed foods and healthier fats. Replacing harmful oils with minimally processed oils such as extra virgin olive oil, coconut oil, and avocado oil, and increasing the intake of omega-3-rich foods can help restore balance and support overall health. Additionally, consumer education and policy changes that promote transparency and nutritional quality are essential for creating a food environment that supports well-being rather than undermining it.

By understanding how dark calories affect our bodies, individuals can make informed dietary choices that promote health and longevity, paving the way for a healthier future.

3) HEALTH IMPACTS OF SEED AND VEGETABLE OILS

Chronic Inflammation: Chronic inflammation is a common outcome of consuming harmful oils. This chapter explains how seed and vegetable oils promote inflammation in the body, leading to a host of chronic conditions, including heart disease, arthritis, and more.

Oxidative Stress and Cellular Damage: Seed and vegetable oils contribute to oxidative stress and cellular damage, which are underlying factors in many chronic diseases. This section discusses the mechanisms of oxidative stress and its implications for long-term health.

Metabolic Disorders and Obesity: There is a strong link between harmful oils and metabolic disorders, including obesity. This chapter examines how dark calories disrupt metabolic processes, leading to weight gain, insulin resistance, and other metabolic issues.

Mental Health and Cognitive Function: The impact of harmful oils extends to our brains as well. This section explores the connection between these oils and mental health issues, including depression, anxiety, and cognitive decline, providing insights into how diet influences brain health.

Chronic inflammation

Chronic inflammation is a significant health consequence associated with the consumption of seed and vegetable oils, primarily due to their high content of omega-6 fatty acids. Omega-6 fatty acids play a crucial role in the body's inflammatory response, serving as precursors for pro-inflammatory eicosanoids. When consumed in excess, particularly in the context of a diet low in omega-3 fatty acids, omega-6 fatty acids can skew the balance towards chronic inflammation.

This persistent immune response involves the release of cytokines, chemokines, and other inflammatory mediators that can damage tissues and disrupt normal cellular function. In the cardiovascular system, chronic inflammation contributes to the development of atherosclerosis, a condition where inflammatory processes in arterial walls lead to plaque formation and narrowing of blood vessels. This process compromises blood flow and increases the risk of heart attacks and strokes.

Within adipose tissue, chronic inflammation contributes to metabolic dysfunction and insulin resistance. Adipose tissue inflammation alters the secretion of adipokines and inflammatory cytokines, disrupting normal metabolic signaling and promoting systemic inflammation. Insulin resistance, a hallmark of metabolic syndrome and type 2 diabetes, is exacerbated by the chronic inflammatory milieu induced by excessive omega-6 fatty acids.

Autoimmune disorders, such as rheumatoid arthritis and inflammatory bowel diseases (IBD), are characterized by dysregulated immune responses and chronic inflammation. The consumption of oils rich in omega-6 fatty acids can exacerbate inflammatory processes in autoimmune conditions, worsening symptoms and disease progression.

At the cellular level, chronic inflammation driven by seed and vegetable oils leads to oxidative stress and cellular damage. Immune cells activated during inflammation, such as macrophages and neutrophils, produce reactive oxygen species (ROS) as part of their defense mechanisms. ROS can damage cellular components, including lipids, proteins, and DNA, contributing to cellular dysfunction and promoting aging processes.

Mitochondrial dysfunction, a consequence of oxidative stress and inflammation, further exacerbates cellular damage and impairs energy metabolism. This dysfunction is linked to neurodegenerative disorders and age-related diseases, where oxidative stress contributes to neuronal damage and cognitive decline.

Balancing the intake of omega-6 and omega-3 fatty acids is essential for mitigating the inflammatory effects of seed and vegetable oils. Omega-3 fatty acids, found in fatty fish (e.g., salmon, mackerel, sardines), flaxseeds, chia seeds, and walnuts, have anti-inflammatory properties that counteract the pro-inflammatory effects of omega-6 fatty acids. Incorporating sources of omega-3 fatty acids into the diet helps restore the balance disrupted by excessive omega-6 intake, supporting cardiovascular health, reducing inflammation, and improving metabolic function.

In conclusion, chronic inflammation induced by the consumption of seed and vegetable oils underscores the importance of dietary choices in maintaining overall health. Understanding the mechanisms through which these oils promote inflammation and contribute to disease pathogenesis informs strategies to mitigate their adverse effects. By prioritizing a balanced intake of omega-6 and omega-3 fatty acids and minimizing consumption of processed foods high in omega-6 fatty acids, individuals can support a healthy inflammatory response and reduce the risk of chronic diseases associated with dietary oil intake.

Oxidative Stress and Cellular Damage

Oxidative stress and cellular damage are critical outcomes associated with the consumption of seed and vegetable oils, particularly those rich in omega-6 fatty acids. These oils, such as soybean, corn, sunflower, and safflower oils, contain high levels of polyunsaturated fatty acids (PUFAs), which are susceptible to oxidation. This susceptibility to oxidation is due to their molecular structure, which includes multiple double bonds that react readily with reactive oxygen species (ROS).

The process of oxidation in PUFAs leads to the formation of lipid peroxides and other reactive molecules within cells. These oxidative byproducts can damage cellular structures, including lipids, proteins, and DNA. Lipid peroxidation, initiated by oxidative stress, compromises cellular membranes and disrupts their integrity and function. This disruption can affect cellular signaling and transport mechanisms, further exacerbating cellular dysfunction.

Proteins, essential for cellular processes, are also susceptible to oxidative damage. Oxidation alters protein structure and function, impairing their ability to perform their intended roles within the cell. This protein dysfunction can disrupt cellular metabolism and contribute to overall cellular stress.

Moreover, oxidative stress can lead to damage in cellular DNA, resulting in mutations and potentially contributing to the development of various diseases. DNA damage induced by ROS can affect cellular replication and repair mechanisms, leading to genomic instability and increased susceptibility to diseases such as cancer.

Mitochondria, the powerhouse of the cell responsible for energy production, are particularly vulnerable to oxidative damage. Mitochondrial DNA, proteins, and lipids can be targets of oxidative stress, compromising mitochondrial function. This dysfunction impairs energy metabolism and reduces cellular energy production, which can have widespread consequences for cellular health and overall physiological function.

Chronic oxidative stress and cellular damage are implicated in the pathogenesis of several age-related diseases and chronic conditions. Conditions such as cardiovascular diseases, neurodegenerative disorders (e.g., Alzheimer's disease, Parkinson's disease), and metabolic syndromes are characterized by oxidative damage to tissues and organs. The cumulative effects of oxidative stress contribute to tissue degeneration, functional decline, and the progression of these diseases over time.

The body possesses antioxidant defense systems to counteract oxidative stress and minimize cellular damage. Antioxidants, both endogenous (produced within the body) and exogenous (obtained from diet), play a crucial role in neutralizing ROS and maintaining cellular redox balance. Enzymatic antioxidants such as superoxide dismutase, catalase, and glutathione peroxidase scavenge ROS and protect cells from oxidative damage. Non-enzymatic antioxidants, including vitamins C and E, flavonoids, and polyphenols from plant-based foods, also contribute to antioxidant defenses and support cellular health.

Dietary choices play a significant role in modulating oxidative stress levels and cellular damage. A diet high in omega-6 fatty acids from seed and vegetable oils, coupled with low intake of omega-3 fatty acids, can exacerbate oxidative stress and increase the risk of oxidative damage to cells and tissues. In contrast, a balanced ratio of omega-6 to omega-3 fatty acids supports cellular health by modulating inflammatory responses and enhancing antioxidant defenses.

In conclusion, understanding the mechanisms through which seed and vegetable oils contribute to oxidative stress and cellular damage highlights the importance of dietary strategies for maintaining optimal health. By promoting a balanced intake of omega-6 and omega-3 fatty acids, incorporating antioxidant-rich foods into the diet, and minimizing consumption of processed foods high in omega-6 fatty acids, individuals can support cellular health, reduce oxidative stress, and mitigate the risk of chronic diseases associated with dietary oil intake.

Metabolic disorders and obesity

Metabolic disorders and obesity are significant health concerns associated with the consumption of seed and vegetable oils, particularly those high in omega-6 fatty acids. These oils, commonly used in processed foods and cooking, have been implicated in disrupting metabolic processes and contributing to weight gain.

The imbalance between omega-6 and omega-3 fatty acids in the diet, with an excess of omega-6 fatty acids from oils like soybean, corn, and sunflower oils, plays a pivotal role in metabolic dysfunction. Omega-6 fatty acids, when consumed in abundance, promote inflammation and insulin resistance. Insulin resistance impairs the body's ability to effectively regulate blood sugar levels, leading to elevated glucose levels over time and increasing the risk of developing type 2 diabetes.

Adipose tissue, which serves as an active endocrine organ involved in hormone regulation and energy storage, is significantly affected by the consumption of omega-6 fatty acids. These oils contribute to adipose tissue inflammation and dysfunction. Excessive intake of omega-6 fatty acids triggers the release of pro-inflammatory cytokines and adipokines from adipose tissue, perpetuating systemic inflammation and metabolic disturbances. Chronic inflammation within adipose tissue not only promotes insulin resistance but also disrupts lipid metabolism, potentially leading to abnormal fat deposition and contributing to obesity.

Research suggests a correlation between the consumption of seed and vegetable oils and increased prevalence of obesity. Diets high in omega-6 fatty acids from these oils, combined with sedentary lifestyles, create an imbalance in energy intake and expenditure, contributing to weight gain. Obesity, characterized by excessive accumulation of body fat, is influenced by genetic, environmental, and dietary factors. Chronic consumption of oils rich in omega-6 fatty acids exacerbates metabolic dysregulation and contributes to obesity-related complications such as cardiovascular diseases, fatty liver disease, and hypertension.

Metabolic syndrome, a cluster of conditions including central obesity, elevated blood pressure, high blood sugar levels, abnormal lipid levels, and insulin resistance, is strongly associated with the consumption of omega-6 fatty acids from seed and vegetable oils. These oils promote inflammation and insulin resistance, contributing to the pathogenesis of metabolic syndrome and increasing the risk of cardiovascular diseases, stroke, and type 2 diabetes.

Balancing the intake of omega-6 and omega-3 fatty acids is crucial for mitigating the metabolic effects of seed and vegetable oils. Omega-3 fatty acids, found in fatty fish (e.g., salmon, mackerel, sardines), flaxseeds, chia seeds, and walnuts, possess anti-inflammatory properties and support metabolic health. Incorporating these sources of omega-3 fatty acids into the diet helps counteract the pro-inflammatory effects of omega-6 fatty acids and enhances insulin sensitivity.

In conclusion, understanding the impact of seed and vegetable oils on metabolic disorders and obesity highlights the importance of dietary choices in maintaining metabolic health. By reducing the consumption of oils high in omega-6 fatty acids, increasing intake of omega-3 fatty acids, and emphasizing whole foods rich in nutrients and antioxidants, individuals can support metabolic function and reduce the risk of chronic diseases associated with dietary oil intake.

Mental Health and Cognitive Function

Seed and vegetable oils, particularly those abundant in omega-6 fatty acids, exert significant influences on mental health and cognitive function. These oils, commonly found in diets rich in processed foods and cooking oils like soybean, corn, and sunflower oils, are increasingly recognized for their potential impacts on brain health.

Omega-6 fatty acids serve as precursors to pro-inflammatory mediators in the body, including cytokines and prostaglandins. When consumed excessively, these fatty acids can contribute to chronic low-grade inflammation, which extends to the brain. Inflammation within the brain has been linked to various mental health disorders, such as depression, anxiety, and cognitive decline. Elevated levels of inflammatory markers are often observed in individuals with these conditions, suggesting a plausible connection between the dietary intake of omega-6 fatty acids and brain inflammation.

Moreover, diets high in omega-6 fatty acids and low in omega-3 fatty acids have been associated with compromised cognitive function and increased vulnerability to cognitive decline with age. Omega-3 fatty acids, abundant in sources like fatty fish, flaxseeds, and walnuts, possess anti-inflammatory properties that counteract the inflammatory effects of omega-6 fatty acids and support optimal brain health. Maintaining a balanced ratio of omega-6 to omega-3 fatty acids is crucial for preserving cognitive function and protecting against neurodegenerative diseases, including Alzheimer's disease.

Research also suggests a correlation between high intake of omega-6 fatty acids from seed and vegetable oils and an elevated prevalence of mood disorders. Conditions such as depression and anxiety may be exacerbated by chronic inflammation triggered by excessive omega-6 intake. Imbalances in neurotransmitter function, particularly serotonin and dopamine regulation, are implicated in mood disorders influenced by inflammatory processes associated with omega-6 fatty acid consumption.

Furthermore, omega-6 fatty acids play a role in influencing neuroplasticity—the brain's capacity to adapt and reorganize itself in response to experiences and environmental changes. During critical periods of brain development, imbalances in omega-6 and omega-3 fatty acid intake can affect neuroplasticity and neuronal connectivity, potentially impacting cognitive function later in life. Adequate consumption of omega-3 fatty acids supports neuroplasticity and enhances cognitive abilities, while excessive omega-6 fatty acid intake may compromise these processes.

Balancing the intake of omega-6 and omega-3 fatty acids through dietary adjustments is crucial for supporting mental health and cognitive function. Increasing consumption of foods rich in omega-3 fatty acids, such as fatty fish, flaxseeds, chia seeds, and walnuts, while reducing the consumption of oils high in omega-6 fatty acids, can help maintain a favorable omega-6 to omega-3 ratio. This dietary approach supports brain health by reducing inflammation, promoting neurotransmitter balance, and enhancing cognitive resilience.

In conclusion, the impact of seed and vegetable oils rich in omega-6 fatty acids on mental health and cognitive function underscores the importance of dietary choices in maintaining brain health throughout life. By adopting dietary strategies that prioritize omega-3 fatty acids and minimize intake of omega-6 fatty acids from processed foods and cooking oils, individuals can support mental well-being, improve mood stability, and reduce the risk of cognitive decline associated with aging and inflammation.

4) THE DECEPTION OF 'HEALTHY' OILS

Myths vs. Facts: The promotion of seed and vegetable oils as healthy alternatives is based on a series of myths. This chapter debunks common misconceptions about these oils, contrasting them with scientific facts to reveal the truth about their health effects.

Marketing Tactics and Misleading Health Claims: The food industry uses various marketing tactics to promote harmful oils. This section examines these tactics, including misleading health claims, to show how consumers are deceived into believing that these oils are beneficial.

Financial Interests and Industry Influence: Financial interests play a significant role in the promotion of seed and vegetable oils. This chapter explores how industry influence shapes scientific research, public policy, and consumer behavior, often at the expense of public health.

Myths vs. Facts

The promotion of seed and vegetable oils as 'healthy' options has been prevalent in dietary advice and marketing for decades. However, several misconceptions exist around their health benefits versus the realities of their impact on human health.

Myth: Seed and vegetable oils are heart-healthy.

Fact: While some vegetable oils, like olive oil and avocado oil, have beneficial properties due to their monounsaturated fats, many seed oils (e.g., soybean, corn, sunflower) are high in omega-6 polyunsaturated fats. Excessive consumption of omega-6 fatty acids relative to omega-3 fatty acids can promote inflammation and contribute to cardiovascular disease risk.

Myth: Seed oils are necessary for a balanced diet.

Fact: While fats are essential for health, the types of fats consumed matter significantly. A balanced diet includes a variety of fats, with an emphasis on monounsaturated and omega-3 fatty acids over omega-6 polyunsaturated fats found abundantly in seed oils.

Myth: Seed oils are natural and therefore healthier.

Fact: The extraction and refining processes involved in producing seed oils often use high heat and chemical solvents, which can degrade the oil's nutritional quality and introduce harmful compounds. Consuming oils in their less processed forms, such as cold-pressed or minimally refined, preserves more of their natural nutrients and beneficial compounds.

Myth: Seed oils lower cholesterol and are therefore good for heart health.

Fact: While seed oils may lower LDL cholesterol levels, they can also decrease HDL cholesterol levels, which is not beneficial for overall cardiovascular health. Moreover, the focus on cholesterol levels alone does not capture the comprehensive impact of oils on heart health, including inflammation and oxidative stress.

Myth: All vegetable oils are equivalent in health benefits.

Fact: Different vegetable oils vary significantly in their fatty acid composition and nutritional profiles. For instance, olive oil and coconut oil, which are predominantly composed of monounsaturated and saturated fats respectively, offer different health benefits compared to polyunsaturated seed oils.

Myth: Seed oils are safe for high-temperature cooking.

Fact: Polyunsaturated fats found in seed oils are more susceptible to oxidation when exposed to high temperatures, leading to the formation of harmful compounds that may contribute to oxidative stress and inflammation in the body. Choosing oils with higher smoke points, such as avocado oil or ghee, can be safer options for high-temperature cooking.

Myth: The benefits of seed oils outweigh their potential risks.

Fact: While seed oils provide essential fatty acids, the overconsumption of omega-6 fatty acids relative to omega-3 fatty acids can disrupt the body's inflammatory balance and contribute to chronic diseases such as cardiovascular disease, obesity, and metabolic syndrome. Balancing intake and choosing healthier fat sources can mitigate these risks.

In conclusion, understanding the myths and facts surrounding the consumption of seed and vegetable oils is crucial for making informed dietary choices. While oils play a role in a balanced diet, prioritizing healthier options and moderation can support overall health and reduce the risk of chronic diseases associated with excessive omega-6 intake.

Marketing Tactics and Misleading Health Claims

Seed and vegetable oils are often marketed as healthy choices, emphasizing specific health benefits such as cholesterol reduction and essential fatty acids content. These claims are frequently based on selective interpretations of scientific studies or industry-funded research, which may not fully represent the oils' overall impact on health. For example, while omega-6 fatty acids are necessary for health, excessive intake relative to omega-3 fatty acids can promote inflammation and contribute to chronic diseases like cardiovascular conditions and metabolic disorders.

Manufacturers often use terms like 'natural,' 'pure,' or 'cold-pressed' to imply minimal processing and healthfulness. However, the production of seed oils typically involves high heat, chemical solvents, and deodorization processes, which can compromise their nutritional quality and introduce harmful compounds. Labels and marketing that emphasize high smoke points may mislead consumers into believing these oils are safe for high-temperature cooking. In reality, polyunsaturated seed oils like soybean or corn oil can oxidize at high temperatures, leading to the formation of toxic by-products that may pose health risks.

Claims of improving heart health through LDL cholesterol reduction are common in marketing campaigns for seed oils. While some oils may lower LDL cholesterol levels, they can also decrease HDL cholesterol levels and affect overall lipid profiles unfavorably. This selective messaging can mislead consumers about the oils' true impact on cardiovascular health. Moreover, the complex nature of nutritional science and conflicting information can confuse consumers trying to make informed choices. Misleading health claims and marketing tactics may contribute to uncertainty about which oils genuinely support health, potentially leading to unintended dietary consequences.

In conclusion, while seed and vegetable oils can be part of a balanced diet, consumers should approach marketing claims critically. Understanding the broader nutritional context and potential health implications of seed oil consumption can help individuals make informed choices that support overall well-being and minimize risks associated with excessive intake of omega-6 fatty acids and processed oils.

Financial Interests and Industry Influence

Financial interests and industry influence exert a substantial impact on the perception and promotion of seed and vegetable oils as purportedly 'healthy' choices in dietary recommendations and consumer marketing. These influences span from agricultural production and scientific research to lobbying efforts and public policy advocacy, shaping both consumer perceptions and governmental dietary guidelines.

One significant aspect of industry influence lies in the sponsorship of scientific research. Seed and vegetable oil industries frequently fund studies that investigate the health effects of their products. While research is crucial for advancing knowledge, studies funded by industry stakeholders may introduce biases. There is a tendency for these studies to emphasize the positive health aspects of oils, such as their essential fatty acid content or potential cholesterol-lowering effects, while downplaying or omitting evidence that suggests adverse health outcomes associated with high omega-6 intake. This selective reporting can skew public perception and contribute to the perpetuation of myths about the health benefits of these oils.

Moreover, industry influence extends beyond scientific research to include lobbying efforts aimed at influencing public policy. Seed and vegetable oil producers engage in lobbying activities to shape government regulations and dietary guidelines that affect their market and consumer perception. By advocating for favorable policies and regulations, these industries can influence the inclusion of their products in dietary recommendations, despite emerging evidence suggesting potential health risks associated with their consumption. This influence on policy-making processes may not always align with the best interests of public health, leading to discrepancies between scientific evidence and official dietary advice.

In addition to lobbying, industry stakeholders invest heavily in marketing strategies that promote seed and vegetable oils as natural and beneficial for heart health. Advertising campaigns often highlight specific health claims, such as cholesterol reduction or essential fatty acid content, to appeal to health-conscious consumers. These marketing tactics contribute to the widespread acceptance of seed and vegetable oils as healthy alternatives to saturated fats, despite ongoing debates and evolving research on their health implications.

Transparency regarding financial ties and conflicts of interest is crucial for maintaining trust in nutritional research and public health initiatives. However, disclosures of industry sponsorship and financial relationships in scientific literature and public health communications are not always transparent or readily accessible to the public. This lack of transparency can undermine the credibility of dietary recommendations and contribute to consumer skepticism about the motivations behind health claims associated with seed and vegetable oils.

Consumer advocacy groups and health professionals play a vital role in educating the public about the influence of financial interests on dietary recommendations. By promoting critical thinking and providing evidence-based information, advocates empower individuals to make informed decisions about their dietary fat intake. Encouraging transparency in industry-sponsored research and policy-making processes is essential for ensuring that dietary guidelines prioritize public health over commercial interests.

In conclusion, financial interests and industry influence significantly shape the perception and promotion of seed and vegetable oils as 'healthy' dietary options. Understanding the implications of industry sponsorship, lobbying efforts, and marketing strategies is essential for evaluating nutritional recommendations and making informed choices that prioritize overall health and well-being without undue influence from commercial interests.

PART II: DETOXING FROM TOXIC OILS

This part is dedicated to the detoxification process, helping you eliminate toxic oils from your diet and begin the journey toward healing. It starts by explaining the body's natural detox processes and how diet can support these functions. The chapters provide practical advice on identifying hidden sources of harmful oils, reading labels, and making healthier choices both at home and when eating out. You will learn about healthy oil alternatives, such as olive oil and coconut oil, and discover cooking techniques and recipes that incorporate these beneficial fats. This part also covers essential nutrients, antioxidant-rich foods, and the importance of balancing omega-3 and omega-6 fatty acids to support recovery.

5) UNDERSTANDING DETOXIFICATION

The Body's Natural Detox Processes: The human body has natural detoxification processes that help eliminate harmful substances. This chapter explains these processes and how they can be supported through diet and lifestyle changes to effectively detox from harmful oils.

The Role of Diet in Detoxification: Diet plays a crucial role in supporting the body's detoxification processes. This section provides an overview of dietary strategies that can help eliminate toxic oils from the body and promote overall health.

Common Detox Myths and Misconceptions: There are many myths and misconceptions about detoxification. This chapter addresses some of the most common ones, providing evidence-based information to help readers make informed decisions about detox practices.

The Body's Natural Detox Processes

The body's natural detoxification processes are intricate mechanisms essential for maintaining health and eliminating harmful substances, including toxins from seed and vegetable oils. Detoxification primarily occurs through several physiological pathways, each playing a crucial role in detoxifying and eliminating toxins from the body.

One of the primary organs involved in detoxification is the liver, which acts as the body's main detoxification center. The liver processes toxins by converting them into water-soluble compounds that can be excreted through urine or bile. This process involves two main phases: Phase I and Phase II detoxification pathways. Phase I involves enzymatic reactions that break down toxins into less harmful substances, while Phase II conjugates these substances with water-soluble molecules to facilitate their excretion.

Another important organ in detoxification is the kidneys, which filter blood and remove waste products and toxins through urine. The kidneys play a vital role in maintaining electrolyte balance and regulating blood pressure, making them essential for eliminating water-soluble toxins processed by the liver.

Additionally, the gastrointestinal system contributes to detoxification by eliminating toxins through feces. The intestines play a critical role in absorbing nutrients and water while preventing the absorption of toxins and harmful substances. Adequate fiber intake supports healthy bowel movements, promoting regular elimination and detoxification.

Furthermore, the skin serves as an auxiliary detoxification organ by eliminating toxins through sweat. Sweat glands excrete water, electrolytes, and small amounts of toxins, contributing to the body's overall detoxification process.

The lymphatic system complements detoxification by transporting toxins and waste products to lymph nodes, where they are filtered and eliminated from the body. Lymphatic circulation helps maintain fluid balance and immune function, supporting overall detoxification and toxin removal.

Optimizing the body's natural detoxification processes is essential for supporting overall health and well-being, especially when addressing the impact of toxins from seed and vegetable oils. By supporting liver function through a balanced diet rich in antioxidants, vitamins, and minerals, individuals can enhance detoxification pathways and reduce the burden of toxins on the body. Adequate hydration, regular physical activity, and sufficient sleep also play vital roles in promoting effective detoxification and supporting overall health.

Understanding the body's natural detoxification processes underscores the importance of adopting healthy lifestyle habits and dietary choices that support optimal detoxification. By prioritizing nutrient-dense foods and minimizing exposure to toxins from processed oils, individuals can enhance their body's ability to detoxify effectively and maintain long-term health and vitality.

The Role of Diet in Detoxification

The role of diet in detoxification is pivotal for supporting the body's natural processes to eliminate toxins, including those from seed and vegetable oils. A well-balanced diet rich in nutrients and antioxidants helps optimize detoxification pathways and reduces the burden on organs responsible for processing and excreting toxins.

Diet influences detoxification primarily through providing essential nutrients that support liver function, enhancing antioxidant defenses, and promoting overall metabolic health. Here's how diet impacts detoxification:

Nutrient Support for Liver Function: The liver is central to detoxification, as it metabolizes and detoxifies toxins into less harmful substances. A diet rich in essential nutrients such as vitamins (e.g., B vitamins, vitamin C, vitamin E) and minerals (e.g., zinc, selenium) supports liver enzymes involved in Phase I and Phase II detoxification pathways. Foods like leafy greens, cruciferous vegetables (e.g., broccoli, Brussels sprouts), and citrus fruits provide essential nutrients that aid liver detoxification processes.

Antioxidant Protection: Antioxidants play a crucial role in neutralizing free radicals and reducing oxidative stress caused by toxins. Berries, nuts, seeds, and colorful fruits and vegetables (e.g., berries, spinach, kale, bell peppers) are rich in antioxidants such as flavonoids, polyphenols, and carotenoids. These compounds help protect cells from damage and support overall detoxification by enhancing the body's antioxidant defenses.

Supporting Gut Health: A healthy gut microbiome contributes to detoxification by metabolizing toxins and promoting regular bowel movements. Consuming fiber-rich foods (e.g., whole grains, legumes, fruits, vegetables) supports digestive health and promotes the elimination of toxins through feces. Probiotic-rich foods like yogurt, kefir, and fermented vegetables also support gut microbiota diversity and function, enhancing overall detoxification.

Hydration and Detoxification: Adequate hydration is essential for kidney function and detoxification, as it supports the elimination of water-soluble toxins through urine. Drinking sufficient water throughout the day helps maintain kidney function and promotes the excretion of toxins processed by the liver and kidneys.

Reducing Toxin Exposure: In addition to supporting detoxification through nutrient-rich foods, minimizing exposure to toxins is crucial. This includes reducing consumption of processed foods containing seed and vegetable oils high in omega-6 fatty acids. Opting for organic produce and minimizing intake of additives, preservatives, and environmental toxins can further support the body's detoxification efforts.

Balancing Macronutrients: Maintaining a balanced intake of macronutrients (carbohydrates, proteins, fats) supports overall metabolic health and energy production, which are integral to detoxification processes. Incorporating healthy fats like omega-3 fatty acids (found in fatty fish, flaxseeds, chia seeds) helps balance omega-6 intake and supports anti-inflammatory pathways, reducing the inflammatory burden on detoxification organs.

In conclusion, the role of diet in detoxification is multifaceted, encompassing nutrient support for liver function, antioxidant protection, gut health promotion, hydration, and toxin reduction strategies. By prioritizing a nutrient-dense diet rich in antioxidants, fiber, and essential nutrients, individuals can optimize their body's natural detoxification processes and support overall health while mitigating the impact of toxins from seed and vegetable oils.

Common Detox Myths and Misconceptions

Common detox myths and misconceptions often circulate in popular culture and wellness trends, influencing perceptions about detoxification processes and practices. Addressing these myths is crucial for understanding the realities of detoxification and making informed decisions about health and dietary choices.

Myth 1: Extreme Cleanses and Fasting are Necessary for Detoxification One prevalent myth suggests that extreme cleanses or prolonged fasting are essential to detoxify the body effectively. However, the body's natural detoxification processes, primarily managed by the liver, kidneys, and digestive system, are adept at eliminating toxins without extreme measures. While short-term fasting or intermittent fasting may support detoxification by reducing the body's toxic load, prolonged fasting or restrictive cleanses can lead to nutrient deficiencies and disrupt metabolic balance.

Myth 2: Detox Diets and Products Eliminate Toxins Rapidly Detox diets and products marketed as quick-fix solutions often claim to rapidly eliminate toxins from the body. These diets typically promote specific foods, supplements, or juices purported to cleanse or flush out toxins. However, scientific evidence supporting the efficacy of such products is limited. Most detox diets lack sufficient nutrients and may lead to short-term weight loss due to calorie restriction rather than true detoxification. The body's natural detoxification processes require a balanced diet rich in essential nutrients and antioxidants to function optimally.

Myth 3: Colon Cleanses are Necessary for Detoxification Colon cleansing procedures, such as colonic irrigation or enemas, are promoted as methods to cleanse the colon and remove accumulated toxins. Proponents of colon cleanses claim benefits like improved digestion and enhanced detoxification. However, these procedures can disrupt the natural balance of gut bacteria, cause dehydration, and lead to potential side effects. The colon naturally eliminates waste products through regular bowel movements facilitated by a fiber-rich diet and adequate hydration, without the need for invasive cleansing methods.

Myth 4: Sweat-based Detox Methods Remove Toxins Saunas, steam rooms, and sweat-based detox methods are believed to eliminate toxins through sweat. While sweating is a natural process that helps regulate body temperature and excrete small amounts of toxins like heavy metals, it is not a primary detoxification pathway for eliminating metabolic waste. Hydration and kidney function are more critical for toxin excretion than sweating alone. Regular exercise that induces sweating can support overall health but should not be relied upon as a sole detoxification method.

Myth 5: Detox Foot Pads and Ion Cleanses Remove Toxins Detox foot pads and ion cleanse devices claim to draw toxins out of the body through the feet using special pads or electrical currents. However, scientific evidence supporting these methods is lacking, and any perceived benefits may be attributed to the pads' adhesive properties or the placebo effect. The body's detoxification processes primarily occur in organs like the liver and kidneys, not through the feet or through electrical currents applied externally.

Myth 6: Detoxing Will Lead to Permanent Weight Loss Detox diets or cleanses are often marketed as methods for achieving rapid weight loss and long-term health benefits. While short-term detox programs may lead to initial weight loss due to reduced calorie intake or water weight loss, sustainable weight management requires a balanced diet and regular physical activity. Detoxification is a natural process that supports overall health but should not be equated with long-term weight loss without sustainable lifestyle changes.

In conclusion, debunking common detox myths and misconceptions is essential for understanding the science behind detoxification and adopting evidence-based practices that support overall health and well-being. Instead of relying on extreme cleanses or products marketed as detox solutions, prioritizing a nutrient-dense diet, hydration, regular exercise, and adequate sleep promotes the body's natural detoxification processes effectively. By fostering a balanced approach to health and nutrition, individuals can support their body's ability to detoxify while maintaining long-term wellness.

6) ELIMINATING TOXIC OILS FROM YOUR DIET

Identifying Hidden Sources of Seed and Vegetable Oils: Harmful oils are often hidden in many foods. This chapter helps readers identify these hidden sources, providing practical tips for avoiding them and making healthier choices.

Reading Labels and Understanding Ingredients: Understanding food labels is crucial for avoiding harmful oils. This section provides a guide to reading labels and identifying ingredients that indicate the presence of seed and vegetable oils.

Identifying Hidden Sources of Seed and Vegetable Oils

Identifying hidden sources of seed and vegetable oils is crucial when aiming to eliminate these potentially harmful ingredients from your diet. Despite efforts to reduce consumption, these oils are prevalent in numerous processed and restaurant foods, making awareness and label reading essential practices.

Many packaged foods, including snacks, baked goods, and frozen meals, contain seed and vegetable oils due to their affordability, long shelf life, and high cooking stability. Common sources include salad dressings, mayonnaise, margarine, and pre-packaged sauces.

Reading ingredient labels carefully can help identify these oils listed under various names such as soybean oil, corn oil, canola oil, sunflower oil, and safflower oil. Moreover, processed foods often contain hydrogenated or partially hydrogenated oils, known for their high trans fat content, despite recent efforts to reduce their use.

Restaurant foods, especially fried and fast foods, are significant sources of seed and vegetable oils. These oils are frequently used in deep frying due to their high smoke points, which minimize oil degradation during cooking. Dishes such as french fries, fried chicken, and tempura often contain these oils, contributing to daily intake without obvious indicators on menus. When dining out, asking about cooking oils used and opting for grilled, baked, or steamed options can help minimize exposure.

Understanding these hidden sources empowers individuals to make informed dietary choices, emphasizing whole foods and cooking methods that avoid or minimize seed and vegetable oils. Transitioning to healthier fats like olive oil, coconut oil, avocado oil, or using butter in moderation offers alternatives that support overall health and reduce the risk of chronic inflammation associated with excessive omega-6 intake.

Reading Labels and Understanding Ingredients

Reading labels and understanding ingredients is essential for identifying and avoiding seed and vegetable oils in processed foods, thereby supporting a healthier diet and minimizing the intake of potentially harmful fats.

When navigating food labels, look for specific terms that indicate the presence of seed and vegetable oils. Common oils to watch out for include soybean oil, corn oil, canola oil, sunflower oil, safflower oil, and palm oil. These oils may also appear under generic terms like "vegetable oil" or "hydrogenated oil." Be mindful that even products labeled as "low-fat" or "healthy" can contain these oils as substitutes for saturated fats.

Additionally, check for ingredients related to trans fats, such as "partially hydrogenated oils" or "hydrogenated oils." These fats are often added to processed foods to improve texture and shelf life but are known to increase LDL cholesterol levels and raise the risk of heart disease. Manufacturers may legally claim a product has zero grams of trans fat if it contains less than 0.5 grams per serving, so it's crucial to inspect serving sizes and consumption amounts.

Understanding the order of ingredients listed on labels is also vital. Ingredients are typically listed in descending order by weight, so products containing seed or vegetable oils near the top of the list likely contain more significant amounts. Foods marketed as "natural" or "organic" may still include these oils, emphasizing the importance of thorough label scrutiny.

For individuals with specific dietary restrictions or health concerns, reading labels becomes even more critical. Ingredients like monosodium glutamate (MSG), artificial flavors, and preservatives often accompany seed and vegetable oils in processed foods, potentially exacerbating health issues such as inflammation or digestive problems.

To make informed choices, consider opting for whole foods and preparing meals at home whenever possible. When purchasing packaged goods, prioritize products with simpler ingredient lists and familiar, whole-food ingredients. By becoming adept at reading labels and understanding ingredient nuances, individuals can proactively manage their dietary intake, supporting overall health and well-being while minimizing exposure to harmful seed and vegetable oils.

Practical Tips for Avoidance at Aome and Eating Out

Avoiding seed and vegetable oils both at home and when dining out is essential for maintaining a healthy diet that minimizes the intake of harmful fats. Here are practical tips to help you navigate food choices effectively:

Cook at Home Using Healthy Oils: When preparing meals at home, opt for healthier cooking oils like olive oil, coconut oil, avocado oil, or butter. These oils are lower in omega-6 fatty acids compared to seed and vegetable oils, reducing the risk of inflammation associated with excessive omega-6 intake. Use these oils in moderation and avoid overheating to preserve their nutritional benefits.

Read Labels Thoroughly: When purchasing packaged foods, carefully read ingredient labels to identify seed and vegetable oils. Look for specific terms such as soybean oil, corn oil, canola oil, sunflower oil, safflower oil, and palm oil. Be cautious of products labeled as "low-fat" or "healthy," as they may contain these oils as substitutes for saturated fats. Choose products with simpler ingredient lists and avoid those with hydrogenated or partially hydrogenated oils.

Choose Whole Foods: Emphasize whole, unprocessed foods in your diet, such as fruits, vegetables, lean proteins, whole grains, nuts, and seeds. These foods are naturally free from seed and vegetable oils and provide essential nutrients, fiber, and antioxidants that support overall health. Incorporate a variety of colors and textures to ensure a diverse nutrient intake.

Prepare Homemade Dressings and Sauces: Instead of store-bought dressings and sauces that often contain seed and vegetable oils, make your own at home using olive oil, vinegar, herbs, and spices. This allows you to control the ingredients and avoid unnecessary additives and preservatives.

Be Mindful When Eating Out: When dining out, inquire about the cooking oils used in dishes, especially for fried or sautéed foods. Opt for grilled, baked, or steamed options whenever possible to minimize exposure to seed and vegetable oils. Ask for dressings and sauces on the side to control portions and choose simpler preparations that prioritize whole-food ingredients.

Request Modifications: Don't hesitate to request modifications to dishes when eating out to accommodate your dietary preferences. Ask for substitutions like olive oil instead of vegetable oil for cooking or omitting sauces that may contain seed oils. Most restaurants are accommodating to dietary requests and can provide alternatives upon request.

Educate Yourself About Hidden Sources: Stay informed about hidden sources of seed and vegetable oils in processed foods and restaurant dishes. Be aware of common culprits such as fried foods, baked goods, snacks, and salad dressings. By educating yourself and reading labels attentively, you can make informed choices that align with your health goals.

Plan Ahead and Pack Snacks: When traveling or eating on the go, plan ahead by packing healthy snacks like nuts, seeds, fruit, or homemade energy bars. This reduces reliance on processed snacks that may contain seed oils and ensures you have nutritious options readily available.

By incorporating these practical tips into your daily routine, you can effectively minimize your intake of seed and vegetable oils both at home and when dining out. Prioritizing whole foods, reading labels, and advocating for healthier cooking methods supports overall health and reduces the risk of chronic inflammation associated with excessive omega-6 consumption.

7) HEALTHY OIL ALTERNATIVES

Benefits of Olive Oil, Coconut Oil, and Other Healthy Fats: Not all oils are created equal. This chapter explores the benefits of healthy fats, such as olive oil and coconut oil, and explains why they are better alternatives to seed and vegetable oils.

Incorporating Nut and Fruit Oils: Nut and fruit oils are also healthy alternatives. This section provides information on how to incorporate these oils into your diet, highlighting their health benefits and culinary uses.

Cooking Techniques and Recipes Using Healthy Oils: Cooking with healthy oils can be delicious and nutritious. This chapter offers cooking techniques and recipes that use healthy oils, helping readers make the switch to a healthier diet.

Benefits of Olive Oil, Coconut Oil, and Other Healthy Fats

Healthy oil alternatives such as olive oil, coconut oil, and various other sources of beneficial fats offer numerous advantages over seed and vegetable oils. These alternatives not only provide essential nutrients but also support overall health and well-being through their unique properties and culinary versatility.

Olive Oil: Olive oil, particularly extra virgin olive oil (EVOO), is renowned for its rich antioxidant content, including polyphenols and vitamin E, which help combat oxidative stress and inflammation in the body. It is a staple of the Mediterranean diet, linked to numerous health benefits such as improved heart health, reduced risk of chronic diseases, and enhanced cognitive function. EVOO is ideal for salad dressings, drizzling over cooked vegetables, and light sautéing due to its low to moderate heat stability.

Coconut Oil: Coconut oil is celebrated for its medium-chain triglycerides (MCTs), specifically lauric acid, which exhibits antimicrobial and anti-inflammatory properties. It is a stable oil suitable for cooking at higher temperatures and lends a subtle coconut flavor to dishes. Coconut oil supports immune function, promotes healthy metabolism, and may aid in weight management by increasing satiety and supporting fat burning.

Avocado Oil: Avocado oil is rich in monounsaturated fats, particularly oleic acid, similar to olive oil. It also contains vitamin E and antioxidants that promote skin health and reduce inflammation. Avocado oil has a high smoke point, making it suitable for high-heat cooking methods such as frying and grilling. Its mild flavor makes it versatile for both cooking and salad dressings.

Flaxseed Oil: Flaxseed oil is prized for its high omega-3 fatty acid content, specifically alpha-linolenic acid (ALA), which supports cardiovascular health, brain function, and anti-inflammatory responses. It is sensitive to heat and light, so it is best used in raw applications such as drizzling over salads, blending into smoothies, or adding to dips and sauces after cooking.

Nut and Seed Oils: Nut and seed oils like walnut oil, sesame oil, and hempseed oil offer unique flavors and nutritional profiles. Walnut oil is rich in omega-3 fatty acids, sesame oil adds a nutty taste and is used in Asian cuisine, and hempseed oil provides a balanced ratio of omega-3 and omega-6 fatty acids. These oils are typically used in dressings, marinades, and as finishing oils due to their delicate flavors and lower smoke points.

Incorporating these healthy oil alternatives into your diet provides a range of nutritional benefits and culinary possibilities. By replacing seed and vegetable oils with these healthier options, you can support cardiovascular health, reduce inflammation, enhance flavor profiles in cooking, and promote overall well-being. Whether used for cooking, salad dressings, or as finishing touches, these oils contribute to a balanced diet that prioritizes essential fats and minimizes the risks associated with excessive omega-6 intake from seed and vegetable oils.

Incorporating nut and fruit oils

Incorporating nut and fruit oils into your culinary repertoire adds not only unique flavors but also diverse nutritional benefits, complementing a healthy diet. These oils, derived from nuts and fruits, offer a range of essential fatty acids, antioxidants, and vitamins that contribute to overall well-being when used thoughtfully in cooking and meal preparation.

Almond Oil: Almond oil is derived from almond nuts and is prized for its mild, slightly sweet flavor and high monounsaturated fat content. It is rich in vitamin E, an antioxidant that supports skin health and protects cells from damage. Almond oil has a moderate smoke point, making it suitable for light sautéing, salad dressings, and baking applications where its delicate flavor can shine.

Walnut Oil: Walnut oil is extracted from walnuts and is notable for its distinct nutty flavor and high omega-3 fatty acid content, specifically alpha-linolenic acid (ALA). Omega-3 fatty acids are essential for heart health, brain function, and reducing inflammation in the body. Walnut oil should be used in cold preparations due to its low smoke point, such as drizzling over salads, adding to dips, or incorporating into marinades for a nutty depth of flavor.

Hazelnut Oil: Hazelnut oil, derived from roasted hazelnuts, boasts a rich, buttery flavor profile that enhances both sweet and savory dishes. It contains monounsaturated fats, vitamin E, and antioxidants that support cardiovascular health and promote skin elasticity. Hazelnut oil is ideal for salad dressings, desserts, and baking applications where its distinctive flavor can enhance recipes without exposure to high heat.

Pumpkin Seed Oil: Pumpkin seed oil is pressed from roasted pumpkin seeds and has a deep, rich green color with a robust, nutty flavor. It is high in omega-6 and omega-9 fatty acids, along with antioxidants like carotenoids and vitamin E. Pumpkin seed oil is traditionally used in Central European cuisines for drizzling over soups, salads, and roasted vegetables, adding a unique taste and nutritional boost.

Avocado Oil: While previously mentioned, avocado oil deserves a special mention here due to its versatility and health benefits. It is rich in monounsaturated fats, vitamin E, and antioxidants, offering a neutral flavor that pairs well with a variety of dishes. Avocado oil has a high smoke point, making it suitable for high-heat cooking methods such as frying, grilling, and stir-frying, as well as for use in salad dressings and dips.

Coconut Oil: Coconut oil, derived from the flesh of mature coconuts, has gained popularity for its medium-chain triglycerides (MCTs) and potential health benefits. It has a mild coconut flavor and a high smoke point, making it suitable for cooking at higher temperatures, including sautéing, baking, and frying. Coconut oil adds a subtle sweetness to both sweet and savory dishes and is a staple in many tropical and Asian cuisines.

Incorporating nut and fruit oils into your cooking not only enhances flavors but also provides essential nutrients that support overall health. Whether drizzling over salads, using in marinades, or incorporating into baked goods, these oils offer diverse culinary possibilities while contributing to a balanced diet rich in beneficial fats, antioxidants, and vitamins. By choosing these healthier alternatives over seed and vegetable oils, you can enjoy delicious meals while promoting optimal health and well-being.

Cooking Techniques and Recipes Using Healthy Oils

Cooking with healthy oils such as olive oil, coconut oil, avocado oil, and nut oils not only enhances the flavor and nutritional profile of your dishes but also supports overall health. Understanding the best cooking techniques and exploring diverse recipes allows you to maximize the benefits of these oils while creating delicious and nutritious meals.

Sautéing and Stir-Frying: Sautéing and stir-frying are quick cooking methods that preserve the flavor and nutrients of ingredients while using moderate heat. Olive oil and avocado oil are excellent choices for these techniques due to their medium-high smoke points and robust flavors. Begin by heating the oil in a skillet over medium heat, then add your choice of vegetables, proteins, or grains. Stir frequently to ensure even cooking and flavorful results.

Roasting and Baking: Roasting and baking foods in the oven allows for even cooking and caramelization of flavors. Coconut oil and avocado oil are suitable for these methods due to their higher smoke points and ability to add a subtle sweetness to dishes. Use coconut oil to coat vegetables or potatoes before roasting, or incorporate avocado oil into baked goods for moist texture and a hint of richness.

Grilling and Barbecuing: Grilling and barbecuing meats, seafood, and vegetables impart a smoky flavor while minimizing added fats. Avocado oil and olive oil are ideal for brushing over foods before grilling to prevent sticking and enhance flavor. Marinate proteins in a mixture of oil, herbs, and spices before grilling to tenderize and infuse them with delicious flavors.

Salad Dressings and Marinades: Creating homemade salad dressings and marinades allows you to control the quality of ingredients and avoid unhealthy additives. Olive oil, walnut oil, and avocado oil serve as excellent bases for dressings due to their rich flavors and health benefits. Combine with vinegar, citrus juice, herbs, and seasonings to create versatile dressings that complement fresh salads or act as marinades for meats and vegetables.

Dipping and Drizzling: Use high-quality olive oil, avocado oil, or pumpkin seed oil for dipping bread or drizzling over finished dishes. Create herb-infused oils by steeping fresh herbs like basil, rosemary, or thyme in olive oil for added flavor complexity. Drizzle avocado oil over soups or roasted vegetables just before serving to enhance their flavors and provide a finishing touch of healthy fats.

Recipes Using Healthy Oils:

Mediterranean Quinoa Salad: Combine cooked quinoa with diced cucumbers, cherry tomatoes, feta cheese, and a dressing made from extra virgin olive oil, lemon juice, garlic, and fresh herbs.

Coconut Curry Chicken: Sauté chicken breast in coconut oil with onions, garlic, ginger, and curry powder. Add coconut milk, vegetables, and simmer until tender. Serve over rice or quinoa.

Avocado Lime Dressing: Blend ripe avocado, lime juice, cilantro, garlic, and avocado oil until smooth. Use as a creamy dressing for salads or as a dip for vegetables.

Walnut Crusted Salmon: Coat salmon fillets with Dijon mustard and press into crushed walnuts. Sear in walnut oil until golden and crispy. Serve with a side of roasted vegetables.

Roasted Vegetables with Herb Infused Olive Oil: Toss assorted vegetables (such as carrots, bell peppers, and zucchini) in herb-infused olive oil, salt, and pepper. Roast in the oven until tender and caramelized.

By incorporating these cooking techniques and recipes into your culinary repertoire, you can harness the benefits of healthy oils while creating flavorful and nourishing meals. Experiment with different oils and flavors to discover combinations that suit your taste preferences and dietary goals, ensuring a balanced approach to cooking that supports optimal health and well-being.

8) SUPPLEMENTATION AND NUTRITIONAL SUPPORT

Essential Nutrients for Recovery: Recovery from the damage caused by harmful oils requires certain essential nutrients. This chapter discusses these nutrients and how they support the body's healing processes.

Antioxidant-Rich Foods and Supplements: Antioxidants play a crucial role in detoxification and recovery. This section explores antioxidant-rich foods and supplements that can help mitigate the damage caused by harmful oils.

Balancing Omega-3 and Omega-6 Fatty Acids: A healthy balance of omega-3 and omega-6 fatty acids is essential for overall health. This chapter provides information on achieving this balance through diet and supplementation.

Essential Nutrients for Recovery

When focusing on recovery and overall health, ensuring adequate intake of essential nutrients plays a crucial role. These nutrients support cellular repair, immune function, and overall well-being, especially in the context of transitioning away from diets high in seed and vegetable oils. Here are some key nutrients to consider for supporting recovery and optimizing health:

Omega-3 Fatty Acids: Omega-3 fatty acids, particularly EPA (eicosapentaenoic acid) and DHA (docosahexaenoic acid), are essential for reducing inflammation, supporting cardiovascular health, and promoting brain function. Found in fatty fish such as salmon, mackerel, and sardines, as well as in plant-based sources like flaxseeds, chia seeds, and walnuts, omega-3s help counterbalance the inflammatory effects of omega-6 fatty acids prevalent in seed oils. Supplementation with fish oil or algae-derived omega-3 supplements may be beneficial for those with limited dietary intake of these essential fats.

Antioxidants: Antioxidants such as vitamins C and E, beta-carotene, and selenium play a crucial role in combating oxidative stress caused by free radicals in the body. Seed and vegetable oils high in polyunsaturated fats can contribute to oxidative damage, making antioxidant-rich foods and supplements important for cellular repair and reducing inflammation. Sources include berries, citrus fruits, leafy greens, nuts, seeds, and supplements like alpha-lipoic acid and glutathione.

Vitamin D: Vitamin D is essential for immune function, bone health, and overall well-being. Exposure to sunlight stimulates vitamin D production in the skin, but dietary sources such as fatty fish, fortified dairy products, and supplements are necessary for individuals with limited sun exposure or higher needs. Adequate vitamin D levels support recovery from inflammation and promote overall resilience.

Magnesium: Magnesium is involved in hundreds of biochemical reactions in the body, including muscle and nerve function, energy production, and protein synthesis. It also plays a role in regulating blood sugar levels and blood pressure. Incorporating magnesium-rich foods such as leafy greens, nuts, seeds, and whole grains can support recovery and reduce the risk of metabolic disorders associated with high intake of seed oils.

Probiotics and Prebiotics: Gut health is essential for overall immune function and nutrient absorption. Probiotics, found in fermented foods like yogurt, kefir, sauerkraut, and kimchi, promote a healthy balance of gut bacteria. Prebiotic fibers, found in foods such as onions, garlic, bananas, and asparagus, provide fuel for beneficial gut bacteria, enhancing digestion and immune function. Supplementing with probiotics may also be beneficial for restoring gut health after exposure to inflammatory seed oils.

Zinc: Zinc is crucial for immune function, wound healing, and protein synthesis. It also acts as an antioxidant, protecting cells from damage. Dietary sources of zinc include shellfish, meat, poultry, dairy products, nuts, and whole grains. Supplementing with zinc may be necessary for individuals with limited dietary intake or increased needs due to inflammation or oxidative stress.

B Vitamins: B vitamins, including folate, B6, and B12, are essential for energy production, nerve function, and DNA synthesis. These vitamins support overall metabolism and aid in the conversion of food into energy. Dietary sources include leafy greens, legumes, whole grains, and animal products. Supplementing with B vitamins may be beneficial for individuals with specific dietary restrictions or increased nutrient needs.

Incorporating these essential nutrients into your diet through whole foods and supplements supports recovery from the inflammatory effects of seed and vegetable oils. Consult with a healthcare provider or registered dietitian to determine individual nutrient needs and develop a personalized plan for supplementation that aligns with your health goals and dietary preferences. By prioritizing nutrient-dense foods and targeted supplements, you can optimize recovery, promote overall health, and mitigate the negative impacts of excessive seed oil consumption on your well-being.

Antioxidant-Rich Foods and Supplements

Antioxidants play a crucial role in combating oxidative stress, which is exacerbated by the consumption of seed and vegetable oils high in polyunsaturated fats.

Incorporating antioxidant-rich foods and supplements into your diet can help mitigate cellular damage, support immune function, and promote overall health and well-being.

Berries: Berries such as blueberries, strawberries, raspberries, and blackberries are packed with antioxidants like vitamin C, anthocyanins, and flavonoids. These compounds neutralize free radicals and reduce inflammation, protecting cells from oxidative damage. Berries are versatile and can be enjoyed fresh, frozen, or added to smoothies, yogurt, or oatmeal for a flavorful antioxidant boost.

Dark Leafy Greens: Dark leafy greens like spinach, kale, Swiss chard, and arugula are rich in antioxidants such as vitamin C, beta-carotene, and lutein. These nutrients support immune function, promote eye health, and reduce inflammation. Incorporate leafy greens into salads, soups, stir-fries, or smoothies to increase your antioxidant intake and support overall wellness.

Nuts and Seeds: Nuts and seeds, including almonds, walnuts, sunflower seeds, and chia seeds, are excellent sources of antioxidants like vitamin E, selenium, and polyphenols. These nutrients help protect cells from oxidative damage, support heart health, and reduce inflammation. Enjoy nuts and seeds as a snack, sprinkle them on salads or yogurt, or use them in baking and cooking to add texture and flavor while boosting antioxidant intake.

Colorful Vegetables: Colorful vegetables such as bell peppers, tomatoes, carrots, and beets are rich in antioxidants like vitamin C, beta-carotene, and lycopene. These compounds neutralize free radicals, support skin health, and promote immune function. Incorporate a variety of colorful vegetables into your meals through salads, side dishes, soups, and roasted vegetable medleys to maximize antioxidant benefits.

Herbs and Spices: Herbs and spices such as turmeric, ginger, cinnamon, and oregano contain potent antioxidants and anti-inflammatory compounds. These ingredients not only enhance the flavor of dishes but also provide health benefits by reducing oxidative stress and supporting immune function. Add fresh or dried herbs and spices to marinades, sauces, soups, and stir-fries to boost antioxidant levels and enhance culinary enjoyment.

Green Tea: Green tea is a rich source of catechins, potent antioxidants that protect cells from oxidative damage and promote heart health. Drinking green tea regularly can support immune function, enhance metabolism, and contribute to overall well-being. Enjoy green tea hot or cold, plain or flavored, as a refreshing beverage to increase antioxidant intake throughout the day.

Supplements: In addition to dietary sources, supplements can provide concentrated doses of antioxidants to support overall health. Popular antioxidant supplements include vitamin C, vitamin E, beta-carotene, selenium, and coenzyme Q10 (CoQ10). These supplements may be beneficial for individuals with specific health concerns or those looking to optimize antioxidant intake beyond food sources.

Incorporating a variety of antioxidant-rich foods and supplements into your diet supports cellular health, reduces inflammation, and enhances overall well-being. Aim to consume a colorful array of fruits, vegetables, nuts, seeds, herbs, and beverages like green tea to maximize antioxidant benefits and mitigate the negative effects of oxidative stress associated with seed and vegetable oil consumption.

Balancing Omega-3 and Omega-6 Fatty Acids

Achieving a balanced ratio of omega-3 and omega-6 fatty acids is essential for promoting optimal health and reducing the inflammatory effects associated with excessive consumption of seed and vegetable oils. While both omega-3 and omega-6 fatty acids are essential polyunsaturated fats necessary for various bodily functions, maintaining a proper balance between these two types is crucial for overall well-being.

Understanding Omega-3 and Omega-6 Fatty Acids:

Omega-3 fatty acids, such as alpha-linolenic acid (ALA), eicosapentaenoic acid (EPA), and docosahexaenoic acid (DHA), are found primarily in fatty fish (salmon, mackerel, sardines), flaxseeds, chia seeds, walnuts, and algae. These fats are known for their anti-inflammatory properties and support cardiovascular health, brain function, and immune system regulation.

Omega-6 fatty acids, including linoleic acid (LA) and arachidonic acid (AA), are abundant in vegetable oils (soybean oil, corn oil, sunflower oil), nuts, seeds, and processed foods. While omega-6 fats are essential for cell structure and function, they are pro-inflammatory when consumed in excess relative to omega-3s. This imbalance can contribute to chronic inflammation, cardiovascular disease, and other inflammatory conditions.

Balancing the Ratio:

The ideal ratio of omega-6 to omega-3 fatty acids in the diet is generally recommended to be around 4:1 or lower. However, modern Western diets often feature much higher ratios, ranging from 10:1 to 20:1 or more, due to the prevalence of processed foods and vegetable oils.

Tips for Balancing Omega-3 and Omega-6 Intake:

Increase Omega-3-Rich Foods: Incorporate fatty fish (salmon, trout, mackerel), flaxseeds, chia seeds, hemp seeds, walnuts, and algae into your diet regularly. These foods provide EPA and DHA directly or ALA, which can be converted to EPA and DHA in the body.

Limit Omega-6-Rich Oils: Reduce consumption of vegetable oils high in omega-6 fatty acids, such as soybean oil, corn oil, sunflower oil, and safflower oil. Check food labels and choose products made with healthier oils like olive oil, avocado oil, or coconut oil instead.

Choose Grass-Fed Meat and Dairy: Grass-fed or pasture-raised animals produce meat and dairy products with higher omega-3 fatty acid content and a healthier omega-6 to omega-3 ratio compared to conventionally raised animals fed with grain-based diets.

Avoid Processed Foods: Processed foods often contain high amounts of refined vegetable oils and hidden sources of omega-6 fats. Opt for whole, unprocessed foods whenever possible to reduce overall omega-6 intake and improve dietary balance.

Consider Omega-3 Supplements: If you struggle to consume adequate omega-3 fatty acids through diet alone, consider supplementing with fish oil or algae-derived omega-3 supplements. These can help achieve a more balanced omega-6 to omega-3 ratio and support overall health.

Benefits of Balancing Omega-3 and Omega-6 Fatty Acids:

Maintaining a balanced ratio of omega-3 to omega-6 fatty acids supports:

Reduced Inflammation: Omega-3s help counteract the inflammatory effects of omega-6s, potentially reducing the risk of chronic inflammation and associated diseases.

Heart Health: Omega-3s support cardiovascular function by reducing blood clotting, lowering triglyceride levels, and promoting healthy cholesterol levels.

Brain Function: DHA, in particular, is essential for brain development and cognitive function, potentially reducing the risk of neurodegenerative diseases.

Immune System: Balanced omega-3 and omega-6 intake supports immune system regulation and response to infections and inflammation.

By focusing on a diet rich in omega-3 fatty acids from sources like fatty fish, nuts, seeds, and algae, while moderating intake of omega-6-rich vegetable oils and processed foods, you can achieve a healthier balance of these essential fats. This approach supports overall health, reduces inflammation, and optimizes your body's ability to function at its best.

PART III: HEALING AND RECOVERY

Healing from the damage caused by toxic oils requires a comprehensive approach that includes nutrition, lifestyle changes, and mental well-being. This part focuses on nutritional strategies for recovery, emphasizing anti-inflammatory foods, cellular health, and gut health. It provides insights into supporting antioxidant levels, detoxifying the liver and other organs, and using natural remedies and supplements. Additionally, this section addresses the importance of mental and emotional well-being, offering strategies for brain health, mood management, and stress reduction. Physical fitness and activity are also highlighted, with guidance on exercise, building an active lifestyle, and incorporating yoga and mindfulness practices.

9) NUTRITIONAL STRATEGIES FOR RECOVERY

Anti-Inflammatory Foods: Certain foods have anti-inflammatory properties that can aid in recovery. This chapter highlights these foods and explains how they help reduce inflammation and promote healing.

Rebuilding Cellular Health: Cellular health is crucial for overall well-being. This section provides strategies for rebuilding cellular health, focusing on nutrients and lifestyle changes that support cell regeneration and repair.

Gut Health and Probiotics: Gut health is integral to overall health. This chapter explores the role of probiotics and other strategies for improving gut health, which can enhance the body's ability to recover from the damage caused by harmful oils.

Anti-Inflammatory Foods

Incorporating anti-inflammatory foods into your diet is a cornerstone of nutritional strategies for recovery, particularly when addressing the health impacts of excessive seed and vegetable oil consumption. Chronic inflammation is a common consequence of imbalanced diets rich in omega-6 fatty acids, which can contribute to various health conditions. Choosing foods with anti-inflammatory properties not only helps reduce inflammation but also supports overall healing and well-being.

Key Anti-Inflammatory Foods:

Fatty Fish: Fatty fish such as salmon, mackerel, sardines, and trout are rich in omega-3 fatty acids EPA and DHA. These fats have potent anti-inflammatory effects, helping to reduce inflammation throughout the body. Aim to include fatty fish in your diet at least twice a week to benefit from their protective properties.

Leafy Greens: Dark leafy greens like spinach, kale, Swiss chard, and collard greens are packed with antioxidants, vitamins (such as A, C, K), minerals (such as calcium and magnesium), and phytonutrients. These nutrients help combat oxidative stress and inflammation, supporting overall immune function and cellular repair.

Berries: Berries such as blueberries, strawberries, raspberries, and blackberries are rich in antioxidants like vitamin C, flavonoids, and anthocyanins. These compounds neutralize free radicals and reduce inflammation, protecting cells from damage and supporting cardiovascular health.

Nuts and Seeds: Nuts (like almonds, walnuts) and seeds (such as chia seeds, flaxseeds) are excellent sources of healthy fats, fiber, and antioxidants. They contain alpha-linolenic acid (ALA), which can be converted into anti-inflammatory omega-3 fatty acids in the body. Incorporate a variety of nuts and seeds into your diet as snacks or add them to salads, yogurt, or smoothies for a nutrient boost.

Turmeric and Ginger: Turmeric and ginger are potent anti-inflammatory spices known for their medicinal properties. Curcumin, the active compound in turmeric, has been extensively studied for its anti-inflammatory effects and may help alleviate symptoms of inflammation-related conditions. Use fresh or ground turmeric and ginger in cooking, teas, or smoothies to reap their health benefits.

Olive Oil: Extra virgin olive oil is a staple of the Mediterranean diet and is renowned for its anti-inflammatory properties. It contains oleocanthal, a compound with similar anti-inflammatory effects to ibuprofen. Use olive oil as a dressing for salads, a dip for bread, or for light sautéing to incorporate its health benefits into your meals.

Tomatoes: Tomatoes are rich in lycopene, a powerful antioxidant with anti-inflammatory properties. Lycopene helps reduce inflammation and oxidative stress, supporting heart health and protecting against certain types of cancer. Enjoy tomatoes raw in salads, cooked in sauces, or as a topping for sandwiches and pizzas.

Green Tea: Green tea contains catechins, powerful antioxidants that help reduce inflammation and protect against cell damage. Drinking green tea regularly may contribute to lower levels of inflammation throughout the body, supporting overall health and wellness.

Incorporating Anti-Inflammatory Foods Into Your Diet:

Create Balanced Meals: Build meals around anti-inflammatory foods, incorporating a variety of colors, textures, and nutrients. For example, start your day with a smoothie made with spinach, berries, chia seeds, and a splash of olive oil.

Snack Wisely: Choose nuts, seeds, or fresh fruit like berries for snacks instead of processed foods high in sugar and unhealthy fats. Pair nuts with a piece of fruit or incorporate seeds into yogurt or homemade granola.

Cook with Healing Spices: Use turmeric, ginger, garlic, and other spices liberally in cooking to enhance flavor and provide anti-inflammatory benefits. Make a turmeric-ginger tea or add turmeric to soups, stews, and curries for an extra health boost.

Stay Hydrated: Drink plenty of water throughout the day to support hydration and help flush out toxins from the body. Add slices of cucumber, lemon, or mint to water for added flavor and antioxidant benefits.

By focusing on a diet rich in anti-inflammatory foods, you can support recovery from the effects of seed and vegetable oil consumption, reduce inflammation, and promote overall health and vitality. Incorporate these foods into your daily meals and snacks to optimize healing and enhance your body's natural ability to repair and thrive.

Rebuilding Cellular Health

Rebuilding cellular health is crucial for recovering from the detrimental effects of excessive seed and vegetable oil consumption, which can lead to oxidative stress, inflammation, and cellular damage. Cellular health refers to the optimal functioning and integrity of cells throughout the body, ensuring they can perform their essential roles in maintaining overall health and well-being.

One of the key strategies for rebuilding cellular health is to focus on nutrient-dense foods that provide essential vitamins, minerals, antioxidants, and healthy fats. These nutrients play vital roles in cellular repair, regeneration, and protection against oxidative damage caused by free radicals.

Essential Nutrients for Cellular Health:

Antioxidants: Foods rich in antioxidants, such as berries, leafy greens, nuts, seeds, and colorful vegetables, help neutralize free radicals and reduce oxidative stress. Antioxidants like vitamins C and E, beta-carotene, and selenium protect cells from damage and support cellular health.

Omega-3 Fatty Acids: Omega-3 fatty acids found in fatty fish (salmon, sardines), flaxseeds, chia seeds, and walnuts are crucial for cellular membrane structure and function. EPA and DHA, specific types of omega-3s, support brain health, reduce inflammation, and promote overall cellular integrity.

Protein: Adequate protein intake is essential for building and repairing tissues, including cellular structures. Sources of lean protein such as poultry, fish, beans, and legumes provide amino acids necessary for cellular repair and regeneration.

Vitamins and Minerals: Micronutrients like vitamin A, vitamin D, vitamin B complex, magnesium, and zinc are vital for cellular energy production, DNA synthesis, and immune function. These nutrients support overall cellular health and contribute to optimal physiological processes.

Healthy Fats: Consuming healthy fats from sources like olive oil, avocado, nuts, and seeds helps maintain cell membrane integrity and fluidity. These fats provide essential fatty acids that support cellular communication, hormone production, and absorption of fat-soluble vitamins.

Lifestyle Factors for Cellular Health:

Hydration: Proper hydration is essential for cellular function and overall health. Drinking an adequate amount of water daily supports nutrient transport, waste removal, and cellular hydration, optimizing cellular processes.

Regular Physical Activity: Exercise promotes circulation, oxygenation, and nutrient delivery to cells throughout the body. Physical activity also stimulates cellular repair processes and supports overall cellular health.

Stress Management: Chronic stress can contribute to oxidative damage and inflammation at the cellular level. Practicing stress-reducing techniques such as mindfulness, meditation, and deep breathing promotes cellular resilience and supports overall well-being.

Quality Sleep: Adequate sleep is crucial for cellular repair, regeneration, and immune function. During sleep, the body undergoes cellular detoxification and repair processes, optimizing overall cellular health.

Practical Tips for Rebuilding Cellular Health:

Eat a Rainbow: Include a variety of colorful fruits and vegetables in your diet to maximize antioxidant intake and support cellular protection.

Prioritize Whole Foods: Choose whole, unprocessed foods rich in nutrients over processed and refined options. Focus on nutrient-dense sources of protein, healthy fats, and carbohydrates to support cellular health.

Limit Toxins: Minimize exposure to environmental toxins, pollutants, and chemicals that can contribute to cellular damage. Choose organic and clean products when possible to reduce toxic burden on cells.

Consult a Healthcare Professional: If you have specific health concerns or dietary needs, consult with a registered dictitian or healthcare provider to develop a personalized plan for rebuilding cellular health.

By adopting a nutrient-rich diet, incorporating healthy lifestyle practices, and minimizing exposure to harmful substances, you can support the rebuilding and maintenance of cellular health. Prioritizing these strategies promotes optimal cellular function, enhances overall health, and aids in recovering from the effects of unhealthy dietary habits, such as excessive consumption of seed and vegetable oils.

Gut Health and Probiotics

Gut health is crucial for overall well-being, influencing digestion, immune function, and even mental health. The gut microbiota, composed of trillions of microorganisms, plays a vital role in maintaining a balanced ecosystem within the digestive tract. This ecosystem includes beneficial bacteria that aid in digestion, produce vitamins, and support immune function. When this balance is disrupted—due to factors like poor diet, stress, antibiotics, or illness—it can lead to dysbiosis, where harmful bacteria may proliferate, contributing to digestive issues, inflammation, and even systemic health problems.

Probiotics are live microorganisms that, when consumed in adequate amounts, provide health benefits to the host. They are found in fermented foods like yogurt, kefir, sauerkraut, and kimchi, as well as in dietary supplements. Probiotics help restore and maintain a healthy balance of gut bacteria by promoting the growth of beneficial strains and inhibiting the growth of harmful bacteria. Different strains of probiotics have specific benefits, such as supporting digestion, enhancing immune function, and reducing inflammation.

For instance, Lactobacillus and Bifidobacterium species are commonly found in probiotic supplements and fermented foods. These strains can help improve digestion, alleviate symptoms of irritable bowel syndrome (IBS), and enhance the gut's ability to absorb nutrients. Saccharomyces boulardii, a beneficial yeast, is another probiotic strain known for its ability to support intestinal balance and combat diarrhea, particularly associated with antibiotic use.

Maintaining gut health involves more than just consuming probiotics. A diverse diet rich in fiber from fruits, vegetables, whole grains, and legumes provides prebiotics—indigestible fibers that fuel the growth of beneficial gut bacteria. Prebiotics act as food for probiotics, helping them thrive and multiply in the gut. In contrast, diets high in sugar and processed foods can disrupt the gut microbiota balance, promoting the growth of harmful bacteria and contributing to inflammation and digestive disturbances.

Stress management is also crucial for gut health, as chronic stress can alter gut microbiota composition and function through the gut-brain axis. Practices like mindfulness, yoga, and deep breathing can help reduce stress levels and support a healthy gut environment. Adequate sleep and regular physical activity further contribute to overall gut health by promoting digestion, circulation, and immune function.

When considering probiotic supplements, it's essential to choose strains that align with your specific health goals and conditions, under the guidance of a healthcare provider. Probiotic supplements vary in their composition and potency, so consulting with a healthcare professional can help ensure you select the most appropriate option for your needs.

In summary, prioritizing gut health through a balanced diet rich in fiber and probiotic-rich foods, managing stress, getting enough sleep, and considering probiotic supplements when necessary can support a healthy gut microbiota. This, in turn, enhances digestion, boosts immune function, and promotes overall well-being from the inside out.

10) <u>REJUVENATING YOUR BODY</u>

Supporting Antioxidant Levels: Maintaining high antioxidant levels is crucial for combating oxidative stress. This chapter discusses ways to support antioxidant levels through diet, supplementation, and lifestyle changes.

Detoxifying the Liver and Other Organs: The liver and other organs play a key role in detoxification. This section provides strategies for supporting these organs, helping to enhance the body's natural detox processes.

Natural Remedies and Supplements: There are various natural remedies and supplements that can aid in detoxification and recovery. This chapter explores these options, providing evidence-based recommendations for supporting overall health.

Supporting Antioxidant Levels

Rejuvenating your body through the support of antioxidant levels involves a holistic approach aimed at combating oxidative stress and promoting overall health and vitality. Antioxidants are essential compounds that play a crucial role in protecting cells from damage caused by free radicals, unstable molecules generated through normal metabolic processes and external factors like pollution, UV radiation, and stress. These free radicals can lead to oxidative stress, which is associated with aging and various chronic diseases.

To support antioxidant levels effectively, it's important to incorporate a diverse range of antioxidant-rich foods into your diet. Fruits and vegetables are excellent sources, particularly those rich in vitamins C and E, beta-carotene, and other phytonutrients. Berries, citrus fruits, leafy greens, and cruciferous vegetables are particularly abundant in antioxidants and can be easily incorporated into meals and snacks throughout the day.

Nuts and seeds also contribute to antioxidant intake, providing a mix of vitamin E, selenium, and polyphenols. These nutrients not only support cellular health but also offer additional benefits such as promoting heart health and providing essential fatty acids. Including a variety of nuts like almonds, walnuts, and seeds like chia or flaxseeds can enhance your antioxidant intake.

Herbs and spices are another valuable source of antioxidants and can be used liberally in cooking. For example, turmeric, ginger, cinnamon, and oregano contain potent antioxidant compounds that not only add flavor to dishes but also contribute to overall antioxidant status. Incorporating these herbs and spices into your daily meals can provide a flavorful way to boost your antioxidant intake.

In addition to dietary choices, managing environmental factors that contribute to free radical production is crucial. Limiting exposure to pollutants, cigarette smoke, excessive sunlight, and processed foods high in unhealthy fats and sugars can help reduce oxidative stress. By minimizing these exposures and focusing on whole, minimally processed foods, you can support your body's natural antioxidant defenses.

While dietary sources should be prioritized, there may be cases where dietary supplements are recommended to support antioxidant levels, especially if dietary intake is inadequate or specific health conditions require additional support. It's important to consult with a healthcare provider before starting any supplement regimen to ensure safety and effectiveness.

By adopting a diet rich in antioxidants from a variety of whole foods, incorporating antioxidant-rich herbs and spices, and making lifestyle choices that reduce oxidative stress, you can effectively support your body's antioxidant levels and promote rejuvenation from within. This holistic approach not only enhances cellular health and resilience but also contributes to overall well-being and vitality, supporting your journey towards optimal health and longevity.

Detoxifying the Liver and Other Organs

Detoxification of the liver and other organs is crucial for maintaining optimal health and well-being. The liver, in particular, plays a central role in detoxifying harmful substances from the body through complex enzymatic processes. These processes involve two main phases: Phase I and Phase II detoxification pathways. In Phase I, toxins are broken down into intermediate metabolites, which are then further processed in Phase II to be excreted from the body via bile or urine. Antioxidants and essential nutrients such as glutathione, vitamins C and E, and various B vitamins are integral to supporting these detoxification pathways.

Supporting liver detoxification begins with adopting a nutrient-dense diet rich in antioxidants and phytonutrients. Cruciferous vegetables like broccoli, Brussels sprouts, and kale contain compounds that enhance liver detoxification enzymes. Additionally, foods such as garlic, turmeric, green tea, and berries contribute to antioxidant defenses and support overall liver health.

Hydration is also essential for liver and organ detoxification, as adequate water intake helps flush out toxins and supports kidney function. Drinking enough water maintains proper blood volume, facilitating the liver's ability to eliminate toxins through urine.

Herbal supplements can complement dietary efforts to support liver health. Milk thistle, known for its active compound silymarin, has traditionally been used to protect liver cells and promote bile production. Dandelion root, artichoke leaf, and schisandra berries are other herbs that may aid in liver detoxification by supporting liver function and promoting detoxification processes.

Reducing exposure to toxins and pollutants is another critical aspect of supporting liver health. Choosing organic foods, minimizing alcohol consumption, and using natural household and personal care products can help decrease the toxic burden on the liver and other organs.

Regular physical activity supports detoxification by promoting circulation and lymphatic drainage, which aids in the removal of toxins from tissues. Exercise also contributes to maintaining a healthy weight and reducing inflammation, further supporting liver function and overall health.

Managing stress effectively is important for liver health, as chronic stress can impact detoxification pathways. Practicing stress-reduction techniques such as mindfulness, meditation, deep breathing, and yoga can help mitigate the effects of stress on the liver and promote overall well-being.

Before starting any detoxification program or using herbal supplements, it is advisable to consult with a healthcare provider, especially if you have underlying health conditions or are taking medications. They can provide personalized guidance and ensure that any detoxification methods are safe and appropriate for your individual needs.

In conclusion, prioritizing liver and organ detoxification through a balanced diet, adequate hydration, herbal support, toxin reduction, regular physical activity, stress management, and professional guidance contributes to overall health and vitality. Supporting these natural detoxification processes helps optimize liver function and promotes long-term well-being.

Natural remedies and supplements

Natural remedies and supplements can play a significant role in enhancing the body's ability to detoxify the liver and other organs. These remedies often leverage the healing properties of herbs, vitamins, and minerals that support the body's natural detoxification processes. Incorporating these natural aids into your routine can help boost liver function, enhance detoxification, and improve overall health.

Herbs have been used for centuries to support liver health and detoxification. Milk thistle is one of the most well-known herbs for liver support. Its active compound, silymarin, is known for its antioxidant and anti-inflammatory properties, which help protect liver cells from damage and promote regeneration. Dandelion root is another powerful herb that supports liver function by increasing bile production, aiding digestion, and helping to flush toxins from the liver. Artichoke leaf extract contains cynarine, which enhances bile production and supports the detoxification process. Schisandra berries are revered in traditional medicine for their ability to protect the liver from toxins, improve liver function, and enhance overall vitality.

Nutrient supplements can also bolster the body's detoxification mechanisms. Glutathione, often called the body's master antioxidant, plays a crucial role in detoxification by neutralizing free radicals and supporting the liver's detox pathways. Supplementing with N-acetyl cysteine (NAC), a precursor to glutathione, can help increase glutathione levels in the body. Vitamins C and E are potent antioxidants that protect liver cells from oxidative stress and support the liver's ability to detoxify. B vitamins, particularly B1, B2, B6, and B12, are essential for liver metabolism and detoxification processes. They help convert toxins into less harmful substances that can be easily eliminated.

In addition to herbs and vitamins, certain minerals and amino acids are vital for detoxification. Selenium is a critical mineral for the antioxidant enzymes that protect the liver from oxidative damage. Zinc supports enzyme function and immune system health, enhancing the body's ability to detoxify. Amino acids like methionine, cysteine, and taurine are essential for the synthesis of glutathione, the liver's primary detoxifier.

Incorporating specific foods known for their detoxifying properties can also support the body's cleansing processes. Cruciferous vegetables such as broccoli, Brussels sprouts, and kale are rich in sulfur-containing compounds that enhance the liver's detox enzymes.

Garlic and onions contain allicin and selenium, which help boost glutathione levels and support detoxification. Beets and carrots are rich in antioxidants and beta-carotene, which support liver health and function. Drinking green tea, which is high in catechins, provides antioxidant support and helps protect the liver from damage.

Hydration is fundamental for detoxification, as water helps flush toxins from the body through urine and sweat. Drinking plenty of water, along with herbal teas like dandelion root tea or milk thistle tea, can enhance detoxification. Adding a squeeze of lemon to water can also aid digestion and stimulate bile production, further supporting liver detoxification.

While natural remedies and supplements can significantly aid in detoxification, it is essential to use them thoughtfully. Consulting with a healthcare provider before starting any new supplement regimen is advisable, particularly if you have pre-existing health conditions or are taking medications. They can provide guidance on the appropriate dosages and combinations of supplements that are best suited to your individual health needs.

In summary, enhancing liver and organ detoxification with natural remedies and supplements can effectively support the body's natural cleansing processes. By incorporating herbs, vitamins, minerals, and nutrient-dense foods into your diet, you can boost liver function, enhance detoxification, and promote overall health and vitality. This approach not only supports the body's natural detoxification pathways but also helps maintain long-term well-being and resilience against toxins.

11) MENTAL AND EMOTIONAL WELL-BEING

Foods for Brain Health: Diet has a significant impact on brain health. This chapter highlights foods that support brain health and cognitive function, providing insights into how dietary choices can influence mental well-being.

Managing Mood and Energy Levels: Diet also affects mood and energy levels. This section offers strategies for managing mood and maintaining high energy levels through nutritional choices and lifestyle changes.

Stress Reduction Techniques: Stress has a profound impact on health. This chapter explores various stress reduction techniques, including mindfulness practices, that can enhance overall well-being and support recovery.

Foods for Brain Health

Maintaining mental and emotional well-being is closely tied to dietary choices, particularly those that support brain health. The brain is a highly metabolic organ that requires a constant supply of nutrients to function optimally and maintain emotional balance.

Incorporating foods rich in specific nutrients can support cognitive function, mood regulation, and overall mental health.

Omega-3 fatty acids are essential nutrients for brain health, known for their anti-inflammatory properties and role in maintaining brain structure and function. Fatty fish such as salmon, mackerel, and sardines are excellent sources of omega-3s, particularly EPA (eicosapentaenoic acid) and DHA (docosahexaenoic acid). These fatty acids support neurotransmitter function, improve cognitive performance, and have been linked to reduced risk of depression and cognitive decline.

Antioxidant-rich foods help protect brain cells from oxidative stress and inflammation, which are implicated in neurodegenerative diseases and mood disorders. Berries such as blueberries, strawberries, and blackberries are packed with antioxidants like anthocyanins and vitamin C, which support brain function and may enhance memory and cognitive abilities. Dark chocolate, rich in flavonoids, also has neuroprotective effects and can improve mood by increasing serotonin levels.

Whole grains provide a steady supply of glucose, the brain's primary energy source, which supports concentration and cognitive function. Foods like oats, quinoa, and brown rice contain complex carbohydrates that release glucose slowly, providing sustained energy and promoting stable mood and mental clarity.

Leafy green vegetables like spinach, kale, and broccoli are rich in vitamins, minerals, and phytonutrients that support brain health. They contain folate, vitamin K, and lutein, which are important for cognitive function and may help reduce the risk of age-related cognitive decline. Cruciferous vegetables also contain sulforaphane, a compound that has neuroprotective properties and may help enhance brain health.

Nuts and seeds are excellent sources of vitamin E, an antioxidant that protects brain cells from oxidative damage. Almonds, walnuts, and sunflower seeds also provide essential fatty acids and protein, which support neurotransmitter function and contribute to overall brain health.

Turmeric, a spice known for its anti-inflammatory and antioxidant properties, has been studied for its potential benefits to brain health. Curcumin, the active compound in turmeric, may help improve memory and reduce symptoms of depression and anxiety by enhancing levels of brain-derived neurotrophic factor (BDNF), a protein that supports brain function and mood regulation.

Probiotic-rich foods such as yogurt, kefir, and fermented vegetables support gut health, which is increasingly recognized for its influence on brain function and mental health. The gut-brain axis plays a crucial role in regulating mood, stress response, and cognitive function, highlighting the importance of a balanced microbiome for overall well-being.

Incorporating these brain-boosting foods into a balanced diet can support mental and emotional well-being. It's essential to prioritize whole foods and minimize processed foods high in sugar, unhealthy fats, and artificial additives, which can negatively impact brain health and contribute to mood swings and cognitive impairment. By nourishing the brain with nutrient-dense foods and adopting a healthy lifestyle that includes regular physical activity, stress management, and adequate sleep, individuals can support their mental resilience and emotional balance for overall well-being.

Managing Mood and Energy Levels

Maintaining stable mood and energy levels is crucial for overall well-being and productivity. Various factors, including diet, lifestyle, and stress management techniques, play significant roles in regulating mood and energy throughout the day. Adopting strategies that support emotional balance and sustainable energy can enhance mental resilience and promote a sense of well-being.

The foods we consume have a direct impact on our mood and energy levels. Eating regular meals that are balanced in macronutrients (carbohydrates, proteins, and fats) helps maintain stable blood sugar levels, which in turn supports steady energy throughout the day. Foods rich in complex carbohydrates, such as whole grains, fruits, and vegetables, provide a sustained release of glucose, the brain's primary fuel source. Protein-rich foods like lean meats, fish, eggs, and legumes help regulate neurotransmitters that influence mood, such as serotonin and dopamine.

Omega-3 fatty acids found in fatty fish, flaxseeds, and walnuts have been associated with improved mood and reduced symptoms of depression and anxiety. Antioxidant-rich foods like berries, leafy greens, and dark chocolate help combat oxidative stress, which can affect mood regulation and cognitive function. Avoiding excessive consumption of refined sugars and processed foods helps prevent energy crashes and mood swings.

Stress Reduction Techniques:

Stress management is essential for maintaining balanced mood and energy levels. Chronic stress can lead to fatigue, irritability, and mood disturbances. Implementing stress reduction techniques can help mitigate the negative effects of stress and promote emotional well-being:

Mindfulness and Meditation: Practicing mindfulness techniques, such as deep breathing, guided meditation, or progressive muscle relaxation, can help calm the mind and reduce stress levels. Mindfulness-based stress reduction (MBSR) programs have been shown to improve mood, reduce anxiety, and enhance resilience.

Physical Activity: Regular exercise is a powerful stress reliever and mood booster. Physical activity stimulates the release of endorphins, neurotransmitters that promote feelings of well-being and reduce stress hormones like cortisol. Activities such as walking, yoga, swimming, or dancing can be particularly effective in reducing tension and improving mood.

Healthy Sleep Habits: Quality sleep is essential for mood regulation and energy restoration. Establishing a consistent sleep schedule, practicing good sleep hygiene (such as limiting screen time before bed and creating a relaxing bedtime routine), and ensuring a comfortable sleep environment can support restful sleep and enhance overall well-being.

Social Support: Maintaining connections with friends, family, and supportive social networks can provide emotional support during times of stress. Talking openly about feelings and experiences with trusted individuals can help alleviate stress and promote a sense of belonging and emotional stability.

Time Management: Prioritizing tasks, setting realistic goals, and managing time effectively can reduce feelings of overwhelm and stress. Breaking tasks into smaller, manageable steps and delegating responsibilities when possible can help prevent burnout and maintain a balanced workload.

Hobbies and Relaxation Activities: Engaging in activities that bring joy and relaxation, such as reading, gardening, listening to music, or practicing hobbies, can provide a mental break from stressors and promote a positive mood.

By incorporating these strategies into daily routines, individuals can effectively manage mood and energy levels, enhance emotional resilience, and promote overall well-being. Recognizing the importance of diet, lifestyle choices, and stress management techniques in supporting mental health underscores the holistic approach to maintaining emotional balance and vitality.

12) PHYSICAL FITNESS AND ACTIVITY

Exercise for Detox and Health: Physical activity is essential for detoxification and overall health. This chapter discusses the benefits of exercise and provides tips for incorporating physical activity into your daily routine.

Building an Active Lifestyle: An active lifestyle supports long-term health. This section offers strategies for building and maintaining an active lifestyle, emphasizing the importance of regular movement for detox and overall well-being.

Yoga and Mindfulness Practices: Yoga and mindfulness practices can support physical and mental health. This chapter explores these practices, providing guidance on how to integrate them into your wellness routine.

Exercise for Detox and Health

Physical fitness and regular exercise play integral roles in promoting overall health, including supporting detoxification processes within the body. Engaging in regular physical activity not only enhances cardiovascular health, muscle strength, and flexibility but also contributes to detoxification by stimulating circulation, lymphatic drainage, and sweat production. These mechanisms help eliminate toxins and waste products from the body, supporting optimal organ function and overall well-being.

Exercise for Detox and Health:

Cardiovascular Exercise: Aerobic activities such as running, cycling, swimming, and brisk walking increase heart rate and respiratory rate, promoting circulation and oxygen delivery throughout the body. Improved circulation enhances the transport of nutrients and oxygen to cells while facilitating the removal of metabolic waste products and toxins. Cardiovascular exercise also stimulates lymphatic circulation, which plays a crucial role in removing toxins and immune cell trafficking.

Strength Training: Resistance exercises such as weightlifting, resistance band workouts, and bodyweight exercises build muscle strength and endurance. Increased muscle mass supports metabolic health and improves insulin sensitivity, which aids in regulating blood sugar levels and reducing inflammation. Strength training also enhances detoxification by promoting the breakdown of toxins stored in fat cells and supporting liver function.

Yoga and Pilates: Mind-body practices like yoga and Pilates combine physical movement with breath control and mindfulness. These practices improve flexibility, balance, and core strength while promoting relaxation and stress reduction. Certain yoga poses and sequences, such as twists and inversions, are believed to stimulate detoxification by enhancing circulation, stimulating digestive organs, and supporting lymphatic drainage.

High-Intensity Interval Training (HIIT): HIIT workouts involve alternating between short bursts of intense exercise and periods of rest or low-intensity activity. This form of exercise can boost metabolism, increase fat burning, and improve cardiovascular fitness in a shorter amount of time compared to steady-state cardio. HIIT also promotes detoxification by enhancing oxygen consumption and metabolic efficiency.

Outdoor Activities: Engaging in outdoor activities such as hiking, trail running, gardening, or playing sports not only provides physical exercise but also offers exposure to fresh air, sunlight, and natural surroundings. Spending time outdoors supports mental well-being, reduces stress levels, and enhances mood, which are important factors in overall health and detoxification.

Mindful Movement Practices: Activities like Tai Chi and Qigong incorporate gentle, flowing movements with deep breathing and meditation techniques. These practices improve energy flow (Qi) throughout the body, promote relaxation, and support stress management. By enhancing circulation and calming the nervous system, mindful movement practices contribute to overall health and vitality.

Incorporating a variety of exercise modalities into a weekly routine can maximize the benefits for detoxification and overall health. It's important to choose activities that are enjoyable and sustainable, as consistency is key to reaping the long-term rewards of physical fitness. Consulting with a healthcare provider or fitness professional can help tailor an exercise program to individual needs and goals, ensuring safe and effective participation in physical activity.

By prioritizing regular exercise, individuals can support their body's natural detoxification processes, enhance organ function, and improve overall health and well-being. Physical fitness not only strengthens the body but also contributes to mental clarity, emotional resilience, and a balanced lifestyle conducive to optimal health.

Building an Active Lifestyle

Building an active lifestyle involves integrating physical activity into daily routines and prioritizing movement as a fundamental part of daily life. This approach goes beyond structured exercise sessions to encompass everyday activities and practices that promote movement, flexibility, and overall well-being.

Living an active lifestyle starts with making small, sustainable changes that increase physical activity throughout the day. Simple actions like taking the stairs instead of the elevator, walking or cycling for short errands, and incorporating movement breaks during prolonged periods of sitting can make a significant difference. These activities not only increase daily calorie expenditure but also promote cardiovascular health, muscle strength, and joint flexibility.

In addition to spontaneous physical activity, structured exercise sessions play a crucial role in maintaining an active lifestyle. Engaging in aerobic exercises such as jogging, swimming, or dancing helps improve cardiovascular fitness and endurance. Strength training exercises, like lifting weights or using resistance bands, build muscle strength and enhance metabolism, which is important for maintaining a healthy body composition and supporting bone health.

Yoga and Pilates are popular activities that contribute to an active lifestyle by improving flexibility, core strength, and mental focus. These mind-body practices also promote relaxation and stress reduction through controlled breathing and mindfulness techniques. Regular participation in yoga or Pilates classes can improve overall physical fitness while fostering a sense of inner calm and balance.

Outdoor activities provide opportunities to connect with nature while staying active. Hiking, gardening, playing sports, or simply spending time outdoors encourage movement and exposure to fresh air and sunlight, which are beneficial for both physical and mental well-being. Being in nature has been shown to reduce stress levels, improve mood, and enhance cognitive function.

Building an active lifestyle isn't just about physical fitness—it's also about prioritizing self-care and overall well-being. Adequate sleep, proper nutrition, and stress management are essential components of a balanced lifestyle that supports long-term health. By making conscious choices to incorporate movement into daily routines and engaging in activities that promote physical and mental well-being, individuals can cultivate an active lifestyle that enhances quality of life and promotes lifelong health.

Yoga and Mindfulness Practices

Yoga and mindfulness practices are integral components of a holistic approach to health and well-being, emphasizing the connection between mind, body, and spirit. Yoga, an ancient practice originating in India, combines physical postures (asanas), breath control (pranayama), and meditation to promote flexibility, strength, and relaxation. Each yoga posture is designed to enhance bodily awareness, improve posture, and increase overall physical fitness.

Beyond the physical benefits, yoga cultivates mindfulness—a state of non-judgmental awareness of the present moment. Mindfulness practices, such as meditation and deep breathing exercises, help reduce stress and anxiety by promoting relaxation and mental clarity. These techniques encourage practitioners to observe thoughts and sensations without attachment or judgment, fostering emotional resilience and enhancing overall mental well-being.

Regular yoga practice has been associated with numerous health benefits, including improved cardiovascular function, reduced inflammation, and enhanced immune response. The practice of yoga can also aid in managing chronic pain conditions, promoting better sleep quality, and supporting healthy aging by maintaining joint flexibility and muscle tone.

Mindfulness practices complement yoga by deepening self-awareness and promoting inner peace. Mindful meditation techniques encourage focused attention on the breath or a specific sensation, helping to calm the mind and reduce the impact of stress on the body. By integrating mindfulness into daily life, individuals can enhance their ability to cope with challenges, improve concentration and decision-making skills, and cultivate a greater sense of well-being.

Incorporating yoga and mindfulness practices into a regular routine offers a holistic approach to maintaining physical, mental, and emotional health. Whether practiced individually or in combination, these techniques provide valuable tools for stress management, personal growth, and promoting a balanced lifestyle conducive to overall well-being.

13) CREATING A SUSTAINABLE HEALTHY LIFESTYLE

Long-term Dietary Changes: Sustainable health requires long-term dietary changes. This chapter offers strategies for making these changes, focusing on building habits that support lasting health and well-being.

Meal Planning and Recipes: Meal planning is crucial for maintaining a healthy diet. This section provides tips for effective meal planning and offers recipes that support a healthy lifestyle.

Building Healthy Eating Habits: Developing healthy eating habits is key to long-term health. This chapter explores strategies for building these habits, helping readers make lasting changes to their diet and lifestyle.

Long-term Dietary Changes

Creating a sustainable healthy lifestyle involves making long-term dietary changes that prioritize nutrition, balance, and overall well-being. This approach focuses on adopting dietary habits that are not only nourishing but also environmentally conscious and socially responsible. Long-term dietary changes encompass choosing whole, minimally processed foods while minimizing the consumption of processed and refined products.

Transitioning to a sustainable diet begins with incorporating a variety of fruits, vegetables, whole grains, lean proteins, and healthy fats into daily meals. These nutrient-dense foods provide essential vitamins, minerals, and antioxidants that support immune function, promote healthy digestion, and contribute to overall vitality. By emphasizing plant-based foods and reducing reliance on animal products, individuals can reduce their carbon footprint and support sustainable agriculture practices.

Making informed choices about food sourcing is another crucial aspect of creating a sustainable diet. Opting for locally grown, organic produce when possible reduces transportation-related emissions and supports local farmers. Choosing sustainably sourced seafood and ethically raised animal products ensures that dietary choices align with environmental conservation efforts and animal welfare standards.

In addition to dietary choices, creating a sustainable healthy lifestyle involves mindful eating practices that promote awareness and enjoyment of food. Practicing portion control, eating slowly, and savoring each bite enhances digestion and prevents overeating. Meal planning and preparation can help individuals make nutritious choices while reducing food waste and saving time and money.

Maintaining hydration is essential for overall health and well-being. Drinking an adequate amount of water throughout the day supports cellular function, regulates body temperature, and aids in digestion and nutrient absorption. Choosing water over sugary beverages reduces calorie intake and supports dental health.

Physical activity is an integral part of a sustainable healthy lifestyle, promoting cardiovascular fitness, muscle strength, and mental well-being. Regular exercise, such as brisk walking, cycling, or yoga, enhances mood, reduces stress, and supports weight management.

Building a support network and seeking professional guidance from registered dietitians or nutritionists can provide personalized advice and encouragement to help individuals achieve their health and wellness goals. By making gradual, sustainable changes to dietary habits and lifestyle choices, individuals can cultivate a balanced and fulfilling way of living that promotes long-term health, vitality, and environmental stewardship.

Meal Planning and Recipes

Meal planning is a cornerstone of maintaining a sustainable and healthy lifestyle, providing structure and guidance for nutritious eating habits. It involves creating a weekly or monthly schedule of meals and snacks that balance nutritional needs, preferences, and dietary goals. Effective meal planning not only supports health and well-being but also promotes efficiency in grocery shopping, reduces food waste, and encourages mindful eating practices.

Benefits of Meal Planning:

Nutritional Balance: Planning meals in advance allows individuals to ensure that their dietary intake includes a variety of nutrients essential for health. By incorporating a diverse range of fruits, vegetables, whole grains, lean proteins, and healthy fats into meals, individuals can meet their nutritional needs and support overall well-being.

Time and Cost Efficiency: Meal planning helps optimize time spent in the kitchen by streamlining meal preparation and reducing last-minute decisions. By preparing ingredients ahead of time and batch-cooking meals, individuals can save time during busy weekdays and minimize reliance on convenience foods, which are often more expensive and less nutritious.

Reduced Food Waste: Planning meals based on weekly or monthly menus allows individuals to buy only the necessary ingredients, reducing the likelihood of perishable items going unused and being discarded. By using leftovers creatively and incorporating them into future meals, individuals can minimize food waste and maximize resource efficiency.

Support for Dietary Goals: Meal planning can accommodate various dietary preferences and goals, such as vegetarian, vegan, gluten-free, or low-carbohydrate diets. By tailoring meals to individual needs and preferences, individuals can maintain consistency in their dietary choices and support long-term health goals.

Tips for Effective Meal Planning:

Create a Weekly Menu: Start by planning meals for the upcoming week, taking into account breakfasts, lunches, dinners, and snacks. Consider incorporating seasonal produce and rotating favorite recipes to maintain variety.

Prepare a Shopping List: Based on the planned menu, create a shopping list that includes all necessary ingredients. Organize the list by food categories (e.g., produce, pantry staples, proteins) to streamline grocery shopping and ensure that nothing is forgotten.

Batch Cooking: Dedicate a day or evening to batch-cook staple ingredients such as grains, proteins, and vegetables. Preparing components of meals in advance makes it easier to assemble quick and nutritious meals throughout the week.

Include Healthy Snacks: Plan for nutritious snacks such as fresh fruit, yogurt, nuts, or homemade energy bars to satisfy cravings and prevent impulsive snacking on less healthy options.

Experiment with Recipes: Explore new recipes and cooking techniques to keep meals exciting and enjoyable. Look for inspiration from cookbooks, online recipe websites, or culinary blogs that focus on healthy and wholesome ingredients.

Sample Meal Planning Recipes:

Breakfast: Overnight oats with chia seeds, almond milk, and mixed berries topped with a spoonful of almond butter.

Lunch: Quinoa salad with roasted vegetables (bell peppers, zucchini, and cherry tomatoes) dressed with lemon vinaigrette and topped with grilled chicken or tofu.

Dinner: Baked salmon seasoned with herbs and served with a side of steamed broccoli and quinoa pilaf.

Snack: Sliced apple with a sprinkle of cinnamon and a serving of Greek yogurt.

By incorporating meal planning into a regular routine and experimenting with nutritious recipes, individuals can cultivate healthy eating habits that support overall well-being. Planning meals in advance not only promotes nutritional balance and efficiency but also empowers individuals to make informed food choices that align with their health and lifestyle goals.

Building Healthy Eating Habits

Building healthy eating habits is a journey that involves making conscious choices to support overall well-being and nutritional balance. Central to this approach is the concept of balanced nutrition, which emphasizes consuming a variety of nutrient-dense foods. These include plenty of fruits and vegetables, whole grains, lean proteins such as poultry, fish, beans, and tofu, and healthy fats like olive oil, avocados, and nuts. By prioritizing these foods, individuals ensure they receive essential vitamins, minerals, and antioxidants necessary for optimal health.

Portion control is another fundamental aspect of healthy eating habits. It involves being mindful of serving sizes and avoiding oversized portions. Using smaller plates and bowls can help regulate portion sizes, while listening to your body's hunger and fullness cues prevents overeating. This practice supports maintaining a healthy weight and reduces the risk of overconsumption.

Mindful eating complements balanced nutrition and portion control by encouraging individuals to slow down during meals, savor each bite, and pay attention to flavors, textures, and sensations. By avoiding distractions such as screens or work while eating, individuals can better appreciate their food choices and improve digestion. Mindful eating promotes a healthier relationship with food and encourages more conscious decision-making about eating habits.

Hydration plays a crucial role in maintaining overall health. Drinking an adequate amount of water throughout the day supports bodily functions, aids digestion, and helps regulate body temperature. Limiting sugary beverages and opting for water, herbal teas, or infused water with fruits or herbs ensures hydration without unnecessary calories or added sugars.

Establishing a routine of regular meals and snacks is essential for maintaining consistent energy levels and preventing excessive hunger. Planning meals ahead of time ensures balanced nutrition and reduces the temptation to rely on convenience foods that may be less nutritious. Variety in food choices ensures a diverse intake of nutrients and flavors, promoting enjoyment of meals and supporting overall nutritional adequacy.

Cooking meals at home using fresh ingredients allows individuals to control the quality and quantity of ingredients, making it easier to choose healthier options and avoid highly processed foods. Incorporating cultural traditions and personal preferences into meal planning adds variety and enjoyment to the diet while ensuring nutritional needs are met.

Lastly, seeking support from registered dietitians or nutrition professionals can provide personalized guidance and recommendations based on individual health goals and dietary preferences. By staying informed about nutrition guidelines and using reliable sources of information, individuals can make informed decisions about their diet and lifestyle.

Building healthy eating habits is a gradual process that involves making sustainable changes to promote long-term well-being. By focusing on balanced nutrition, portion control, mindful eating, hydration, regular meals and snacks, variety in food choices, cooking at home, and seeking professional guidance, individuals can cultivate a positive relationship with food and achieve their health goals effectively.

PART IV: BEYOND THE KITCHEN

Health and wellness extend beyond dietary choices, encompassing a holistic approach that integrates mind, body, and spirit. This part explores holistic approaches to wellness, including alternative therapies, sleep, and the role of integrative practices in healing. It emphasizes the importance of advocacy and awareness, providing strategies for educating others about the risks of harmful oils and supporting policy changes for healthier food standards. Community involvement and grassroots movements are highlighted as powerful tools for creating lasting change. The final chapters look to the future, discussing emerging research, innovations in food science, and the evolving landscape of dietary guidelines.

14) HOLISTIC APPROACHES TO WELLNESS

Integrating Mind, Body, and Spirit: Wellness goes beyond physical health. This chapter discusses the importance of integrating mind, body, and spirit in a holistic approach to wellness, emphasizing the interconnectedness of these aspects of health.

Alternative Therapies and Practices: There are various alternative therapies and practices that can support overall health. This section explores these options, providing evidence-based information on their benefits and uses.

Sleep and Its Role in Healing: Sleep is essential for healing and recovery. This chapter highlights the importance of sleep and offers tips for improving sleep quality to support overall health.

Integrating Mind, Body, and Spirit

Integrating mind, body, and spirit is central to holistic approaches to wellness, emphasizing the interconnectedness of physical health, mental well-being, and spiritual fulfillment. This approach recognizes that optimal health encompasses more than just the absence of illness—it involves nurturing a harmonious relationship between the mind, body, and spirit to achieve overall wellness and vitality.

Mind: Mental well-being plays a crucial role in holistic health. Practices such as mindfulness meditation, cognitive behavioral techniques, and stress management strategies promote emotional resilience and enhance mental clarity. By cultivating awareness of thoughts and emotions, individuals can develop healthier coping mechanisms and improve their overall mood and cognitive function.

Body: Physical health encompasses maintaining a balanced diet, engaging in regular exercise, and practicing preventive healthcare measures. Physical activity, whether through aerobic exercises, strength training, or yoga, not only improves cardiovascular fitness and muscle tone but also enhances mood and reduces stress levels. Adequate sleep, hydration, and proper nutrition provide essential support for bodily functions and contribute to overall vitality.

Spirit: Spiritual well-being involves nurturing a sense of purpose, connection, and inner peace. Practices such as meditation, prayer, spending time in nature, or engaging in creative pursuits can foster a deeper understanding of oneself and promote spiritual growth. Cultivating meaningful relationships and participating in community activities also contribute to a sense of belonging and fulfillment.

Holistic Approaches: Holistic approaches to wellness integrate these elements—mind, body, and spirit—into a cohesive framework that supports overall health and well-being. By addressing the interconnected aspects of health, individuals can achieve greater resilience to stress, enhance their quality of life, and experience a deeper sense of purpose and fulfillment.

Benefits of Integration: Integrating mind, body, and spirit promotes a balanced and harmonious life. It enhances self-awareness, improves emotional regulation, and supports physical health outcomes such as immune function and longevity. By fostering a holistic approach to wellness, individuals can experience greater resilience to life's challenges, cultivate healthier habits, and nurture a positive outlook on life.

Incorporating holistic practices into daily routines—such as mindfulness exercises, physical activity, and spiritual reflection—can promote overall wellness and contribute to a more fulfilling and balanced lifestyle. By prioritizing the integration of mind, body, and spirit, individuals can cultivate resilience, enhance their sense of well-being, and pursue a path toward optimal health and vitality.

Alternative Therapies and Practices

Alternative therapies and practices encompass a diverse array of approaches that complement conventional medicine in promoting holistic well-being and healing. These modalities often emphasize the interconnectedness of mind, body, and spirit, aiming to address the root causes of health issues and support the body's natural healing processes.

Many alternative therapies draw from traditional healing systems worldwide, such as acupuncture, which involves inserting thin needles into specific points on the body to restore energy flow and promote balance. Traditional Chinese medicine incorporates acupuncture along with herbal remedies, dietary adjustments, and practices like tai chi or qigong to maintain health and prevent illness.

Ayurveda, originating from India, focuses on balancing three elemental energies, or doshas—Vata, Pitta, and Kapha—through personalized diet, lifestyle recommendations, herbal supplements, and detoxification practices. Naturopathy utilizes natural therapies such as nutrition counseling, botanical medicine, hydrotherapy, and lifestyle modifications to stimulate the body's innate healing mechanisms and optimize health.

Chiropractic care emphasizes spinal adjustments and musculoskeletal alignment to alleviate pain, improve mobility, and enhance overall well-being. Homeopathy uses highly diluted substances to stimulate the body's self-healing responses and address underlying imbalances contributing to health conditions. Herbal medicine employs plant-based remedies like teas, tinctures, and extracts to support various aspects of health, from immune function to stress management.

Integrating Alternative Therapies

Integrative medicine combines alternative therapies with conventional medical treatments to create comprehensive, personalized healthcare plans. This approach aims to enhance therapeutic outcomes, improve quality of life, and empower individuals to take an active role in their health and well-being. By addressing the whole person—physical, emotional, and spiritual—integrative medicine supports holistic healing and encourages collaboration between healthcare providers and patients.

Benefits and Considerations

Alternative therapies offer several potential benefits, including reduced reliance on pharmaceuticals, personalized treatment plans tailored to individual needs, and support for chronic conditions or symptoms that may not respond well to conventional treatments alone. These therapies also promote holistic care by addressing underlying imbalances and supporting overall well-being. However, it's essential to approach alternative therapies with an informed perspective, considering safety, evidence-based practices, practitioner qualifications, and potential interactions with existing treatments.

Sleep and Its Role in Healing

Sleep plays a crucial role in promoting healing, supporting overall health, and optimizing daily functioning. Quality sleep is essential for physical restoration, cognitive function, emotional well-being, and immune system regulation. During sleep, the body undergoes vital processes that contribute to healing, repair, and maintenance of bodily functions.

Functions of Sleep

Sleep supports physical restoration by repairing tissues, replenishing energy stores, and promoting muscle growth through the release of growth hormone during deep sleep stages. Cognitive function benefits from sleep through memory consolidation, learning processes, and decision-making abilities. Emotional regulation is also enhanced by sleep, which helps to manage stress and regulate mood through neurotransmitter and hormone balance. Additionally, sleep plays a key role in supporting the immune system by stimulating the production of cytokines and antibodies that protect against infections and inflammation.

Factors Influencing Sleep Quality

Sleep quality can be influenced by various factors, including sleep hygiene practices, environmental conditions, lifestyle choices, and underlying health conditions. Practicing good sleep hygiene involves establishing a regular sleep schedule, creating a comfortable sleep environment, and incorporating relaxation techniques to promote restful sleep.

Tips for Improving Sleep Quality

Maintain a consistent sleep schedule by going to bed and waking up at the same time each day, even on weekends.

Establish a relaxing bedtime routine that includes activities such as reading, gentle stretching, or taking a warm bath to signal to your body that it's time to wind down.

Optimize your sleep environment by minimizing noise, light, and electronic devices that can disrupt sleep. Use comfortable bedding and maintain a cool, comfortable room temperature.

Limit consumption of stimulants like caffeine and nicotine close to bedtime, as they can interfere with sleep. Alcohol should also be limited, as it disrupts sleep patterns and can lead to fragmented sleep.

Manage stress through techniques such as deep breathing, meditation, or progressive muscle relaxation to promote relaxation and improve sleep quality.

Health Benefits of Adequate Sleep

Prioritizing adequate sleep supports overall health and well-being by enhancing physical and mental resilience, improving cognitive function, and reducing the risk of chronic diseases such as cardiovascular disease, diabetes, and obesity. Recognizing the importance of sleep in promoting healing and maintaining optimal health allows individuals to prioritize sleep as an essential component of their wellness routine.

15) ADVOCACY AND AWARENESS

Advocacy and awareness efforts are fundamental pillars in public health initiatives aimed at promoting healthier lifestyles and reducing the prevalence of preventable diseases. These strategies involve educating individuals about health risks associated with dietary choices, lifestyle habits, environmental factors, and advocating for policy changes that enhance food standards. By mobilizing community involvement through grassroots movements, stakeholders can empower individuals to make informed decisions and create supportive environments for health.

Educating Others About the Risks

Educating the public about health risks is essential for raising awareness and empowering individuals to prioritize their well-being. Health education initiatives focus on disseminating evidence-based information through various channels such as campaigns, educational programs, workshops, online resources, and community outreach events. These efforts address key health concerns, including the impact of poor dietary choices, sedentary lifestyles, tobacco and alcohol use, environmental pollutants, and stress on overall health outcomes.

Effective health education campaigns highlight the consequences of unhealthy behaviors, such as increased risks of chronic diseases like diabetes, cardiovascular diseases, obesity, and certain cancers. They emphasize the importance of adopting balanced diets rich in fruits, vegetables, whole grains, and lean proteins, along with regular physical activity and stress management techniques. By promoting knowledge and understanding of these factors, advocacy programs aim to empower individuals to make informed decisions that contribute to their long-term health and well-being.

In addition to individual behavior change, health education also addresses social determinants of health, including socioeconomic factors, access to healthcare services, and environmental conditions that influence health outcomes. By fostering a deeper understanding of these determinants, advocacy efforts can advocate for policies and initiatives that address health disparities and promote equitable access to resources for all communities.

Supporting Policy Changes for Healthier Food Standards

Advocating for policy changes is instrumental in creating environments that support healthier food choices and reduce the prevalence of obesity and chronic diseases. Policy advocacy focuses on influencing legislation, regulations, and institutional practices to improve food standards, nutrition labeling, and promote sustainable agricultural practices. Key policy initiatives include:

Nutrition Labeling and Menu Transparency: Advocacy efforts support regulations that require clear and accessible nutrition labeling on packaged foods and menu items in restaurants. These labels provide consumers with information about calorie content, serving sizes, and nutritional value, empowering them to make informed food choices that align with their dietary preferences and health goals.

Reducing Sugar, Salt, and Trans Fats: Advocates work to reduce the availability and consumption of added sugars, excessive sodium, and trans fats in processed foods and beverages. Policies may include setting limits on these ingredients, implementing taxes or subsidies to incentivize healthier alternatives, and promoting industry reformulation of products to meet healthier nutritional standards.

Promoting Healthy Food Environments: Advocacy efforts support initiatives that create healthier food environments in schools, workplaces, hospitals, and community settings. This includes promoting access to fresh fruits, vegetables, and whole grains, reducing the availability of unhealthy snacks and sugary beverages, and implementing nutrition education programs to promote healthier eating habits among children and adults.

Supporting Sustainable Agriculture: Advocacy for sustainable agricultural practices promotes environmentally friendly farming methods that prioritize soil health, biodiversity conservation, and reduced use of pesticides and synthetic fertilizers. These practices not only support healthier food production but also contribute to environmental sustainability and resilience to climate change.

Community Involvement and Grassroots Movements

Community involvement and grassroots movements play a crucial role in driving sustainable change and fostering a culture of health within local communities. These initiatives mobilize individuals, community organizations, schools, businesses, healthcare providers, and policymakers to collaborate on health-promoting activities and advocate for policies that support healthier lifestyles.

Key Components of Community Involvement and Grassroots Movements:

Health Fairs and Community Events: Organizing health fairs, wellness workshops, cooking demonstrations, and fitness classes engages community members in learning about health-promoting behaviors and accessing preventive health services. These events provide opportunities for education, health screenings, and networking with local healthcare providers and organizations.

Community Gardens and Nutrition Programs: Establishing community gardens and nutrition programs promotes access to fresh, locally grown produce and encourages community members to incorporate more fruits and vegetables into their diets. These initiatives foster food security, support sustainable food systems, and educate participants about gardening skills, nutrition, and healthy cooking methods.

Advocacy Campaigns and Policy Initiatives: Grassroots movements mobilize community members to advocate for policies and initiatives that promote health equity, improve access to healthcare services, and address social determinants of health. Campaigns may focus on issues such as affordable housing, transportation access, economic opportunities, and environmental justice to create supportive environments for health in underserved communities.

School and Workplace Wellness Programs: Collaborating with schools and workplaces to implement wellness programs encourages healthy behaviors among students, employees, and their families. These programs may include physical activity challenges, nutrition education workshops, stress management techniques, and policies that support healthy food options in cafeterias and vending machines.

Digital and Social Media Campaigns: Leveraging digital platforms and social media channels increases outreach and engagement in health advocacy efforts. Campaigns raise awareness about health issues, share educational resources, promote community events, and encourage dialogue among stakeholders interested in improving health outcomes.

Impact of Advocacy and Grassroots Efforts

Advocacy and grassroots movements have a significant impact on promoting healthier lifestyles, influencing policy changes, and addressing health disparities within communities. By mobilizing collective action and empowering individuals to become advocates for their health, these efforts contribute to building resilient communities where everyone has the opportunity to thrive.

Challenges and Considerations

While advocacy and grassroots movements play a critical role in promoting public health initiatives, they also face challenges and considerations that impact their effectiveness and sustainability:

Resource Mobilization: Securing funding, resources, and support from stakeholders is essential for sustaining advocacy efforts and implementing community-based initiatives. Collaboration with local governments, nonprofit organizations, businesses, and philanthropic foundations can strengthen advocacy campaigns and expand their reach.

Building Partnerships: Establishing partnerships and collaborations with diverse stakeholders, including healthcare providers, policymakers, community leaders, educators, and businesses, enhances the impact and credibility of advocacy efforts. These partnerships facilitate information sharing, resource pooling, and collective problem-solving to address complex health challenges.

Addressing Health Inequities: Advocacy efforts must prioritize addressing health inequities and disparities that disproportionately affect marginalized and underserved populations. This requires advocating for policies and interventions that promote health equity, improve access to healthcare services, and address social determinants of health such as poverty, discrimination, and environmental injustice.

Cultural Competence: Recognizing and respecting cultural diversity, beliefs, and practices within communities is essential for effectively engaging stakeholders in advocacy and grassroots movements. Cultural competence ensures that health messages are culturally appropriate, accessible, and inclusive, promoting trust and participation among diverse populations.

Monitoring and Evaluation: Continuous monitoring and evaluation of advocacy efforts and community-based initiatives are critical for measuring impact, identifying areas for improvement, and informing strategic decision-making. Collecting data on health outcomes, behavior change, and community engagement allows advocates to demonstrate success, leverage support, and advocate for sustained investment in public health.

Advocacy and awareness efforts, supported by community involvement and grassroots movements, are instrumental in promoting public health, influencing policy changes, and fostering environments that support healthier lifestyles. By educating individuals about health risks, advocating for policies that improve food standards, and mobilizing communities to take collective action, stakeholders can empower individuals to make informed decisions and create sustainable changes that enhance overall health and well-being.

Through collaborative efforts, stakeholders can address health disparities, promote health equity, and build resilient communities where everyone has the opportunity to lead healthier, more fulfilling lives. Advocacy and grassroots movements continue to play a crucial role in shaping the future of public health by advocating for policies that support healthier lifestyles and create supportive environments for health within communities.

16) RESEARCH AND FUTURE DIRECTIONS

Research and future directions in public health and nutrition are crucial for advancing scientific knowledge, identifying emerging trends, and shaping future dietary guidelines. This section explores emerging studies and trends, innovations in food science and nutrition, and the evolving landscape of dietary guidelines to address contemporary health challenges and promote optimal well-being.

Emerging Studies and Trends

Emerging studies in nutrition and public health research are exploring novel areas to better understand the impact of diet on health outcomes, disease prevention, and overall well-being. Recent trends highlight advancements in nutritional epidemiology, personalized nutrition, and the microbiome's role in health.

Nutritional Epidemiology: Advancements in nutritional epidemiology are shedding light on the complex relationships between dietary patterns, nutrient intake, and chronic diseases. Longitudinal studies and meta-analyses are providing insights into the effects of specific nutrients, foods, and dietary patterns on health outcomes such as cardiovascular disease, diabetes, obesity, and cancer.

Personalized Nutrition: The concept of personalized nutrition is gaining traction, aiming to tailor dietary recommendations based on individual genetic profiles, metabolic factors, and lifestyle preferences. Advances in genomic research and digital health technologies enable personalized nutrition interventions that optimize health outcomes and improve dietary adherence among diverse populations.

Microbiome Research: Research on the gut microbiome's influence on health is expanding our understanding of how microbial communities interact with dietary components to impact immune function, metabolism, and disease susceptibility. Emerging studies explore the role of probiotics, prebiotics, and dietary fibers in promoting gut health and mitigating chronic inflammatory conditions.

Impact of Environmental Factors: Studies are investigating the impact of environmental factors, such as climate change, food production practices, and food insecurity, on global nutrition and public health. Research in sustainable food systems, food security interventions, and the environmental footprint of dietary choices aims to promote environmentally sustainable diets that support human health and planetary health.

Innovations in Food Science and Nutrition

Innovations in food science and nutrition are driving advancements in food production, processing technologies, and nutritional quality to meet evolving consumer preferences and health needs. These innovations encompass functional foods, alternative protein sources, food fortification, and sustainable food packaging solutions.

Functional Foods: Functional foods are enriched with bioactive compounds, vitamins, minerals, and antioxidants that offer potential health benefits beyond basic nutrition. Innovations in functional food development include fortified dairy products, plant-based beverages, fortified cereals, and nutritional supplements targeted at improving specific health outcomes, such as cardiovascular health, digestive health, and cognitive function.

Alternative Protein Sources: The growing demand for sustainable protein sources has led to innovations in alternative protein production, including plant-based proteins (e.g., soy, pea, and lentil proteins), cultured meat, algae-based proteins, and insect-derived proteins. These alternative protein sources offer environmental benefits, reduce reliance on animal agriculture, and provide nutritious alternatives for individuals adopting plant-based diets.

Food Fortification: Food fortification involves adding essential nutrients, such as vitamins (e.g., vitamin D, folic acid, vitamin B12) and minerals (e.g., iron, zinc, iodine), to staple foods and processed products to address nutrient deficiencies and improve public health outcomes. Innovations in food fortification technologies ensure the stability, bioavailability, and sensory acceptability of fortified foods, supporting global efforts to combat malnutrition and promote micronutrient adequacy.

Sustainable Food Packaging: Innovations in sustainable food packaging aim to reduce food waste, minimize environmental impact, and enhance food safety during storage and transportation. Biodegradable materials, compostable packaging, recyclable plastics, and active packaging technologies (e.g., antimicrobial films, oxygen scavengers) improve shelf life, preserve food quality, and support sustainable consumption practices.

The Future of Dietary Guidelines

The future of dietary guidelines is evolving to reflect advances in nutrition science, dietary patterns, cultural diversity, and global health challenges. Updated guidelines emphasize holistic approaches to health promotion, sustainability, and equitable access to nutritious foods.

Holistic Health Approaches: Future dietary guidelines integrate holistic health approaches that consider the interplay between diet, physical activity, sleep, stress management, and mental well-being. Recommendations prioritize whole-food-based diets, plant-forward eating patterns, and mindful eating practices that support overall health and longevity.

Sustainability and Environmental Impact: Dietary guidelines increasingly emphasize sustainable food choices and environmentally responsible dietary patterns that reduce greenhouse gas emissions, conserve natural resources, and promote biodiversity. Recommendations encourage consumption of locally sourced foods, plant-based proteins, and minimally processed foods to support planetary health and mitigate climate change.

Cultural and Ethnic Diversity: Recognizing cultural and ethnic diversity in dietary habits, future guidelines incorporate culturally appropriate nutrition recommendations that respect traditional diets, culinary practices, and food customs. Tailored dietary advice considers dietary preferences, food access barriers, and community-specific health needs to promote dietary inclusivity and improve health outcomes across diverse populations.

Evidence-Based Policy Recommendations: Evidence-based policy recommendations support the implementation of dietary guidelines through collaborations between public health authorities, policymakers, healthcare providers, educators, and food industry stakeholders. Strategies include nutrition education programs, food labeling initiatives, fiscal policies (e.g., taxation, subsidies), and regulatory measures that create supportive environments for healthy eating behaviors and sustainable food systems.

Research and future directions in public health and nutrition are critical for advancing scientific knowledge, addressing emerging health challenges, and shaping evidence-based dietary guidelines that promote optimal health outcomes for individuals and populations worldwide. Innovations in food science, personalized nutrition, and sustainable food systems drive advancements in dietary recommendations, food production practices, and public health policies aimed at improving dietary quality, reducing disease burden, and enhancing global health equity.

By leveraging research insights, fostering technological innovations, and advocating for evidence-based policy changes, stakeholders can contribute to building healthier, more resilient communities and sustainable food systems that support human health, environmental sustainability, and social well-being in the years to come.

CONCLUSION

In conclusion, "Dark Calories and Toxic Oils Detox for Healthy Healing" has explored key findings that underscore the profound impact of seed oils and vegetable oils on human health, while providing actionable insights for detoxification and achieving overall wellness.

Throughout the book, we uncovered the historical rise of vegetable oils and their pervasive influence on dietary guidelines, revealing how these oils, once touted as beneficial, contribute to a spectrum of health issues. We defined "dark calories" as a concept encapsulating the hidden harm of these oils, which promote chronic inflammation, oxidative stress, and metabolic disorders within the body. By understanding the biochemical mechanisms behind their detrimental effects, readers gained clarity on why these oils pose such a significant risk to health.

A critical aspect addressed was the deception surrounding "healthy" oils, where myths versus facts were dismantled to reveal the misleading marketing tactics used by the industry. Financial interests and industry influence were exposed, highlighting how these factors perpetuate misconceptions about the health benefits of seed and vegetable oils. Armed with this knowledge, readers learned to discern and identify hidden sources of these oils in everyday foods, empowering them to make informed dietary choices.

The book emphasized the importance of eliminating toxic oils from one's diet and replacing them with healthier alternatives such as olive oil and coconut oil. Practical tips for avoidance at home and when eating out were provided, ensuring readers could navigate their food choices with confidence. Additionally, strategies for balancing omega-3 and omega-6 fatty acids, along with the role of antioxidants and essential nutrients in supporting recovery, were detailed to promote cellular health and overall well-being.

Beyond dietary considerations, the book advocated for a holistic approach to healing and recovery. It addressed the significance of gut health and probiotics, offered insights into natural remedies and supplements, and explored mental and emotional well-being through foods for brain health, stress management techniques, and mindfulness practices. Physical fitness and active lifestyle habits were also encouraged as integral components of a sustainable healthy lifestyle.

Looking forward, the future of dietary guidelines was discussed in light of emerging studies and trends in nutrition science. Innovations in food science and sustainable food systems were highlighted as pivotal for shaping evidence-based dietary recommendations and promoting environmental sustainability. The book concluded with a call to action, urging readers to advocate for healthier food standards, educate others about the risks of toxic oils, and engage in community-driven initiatives that support holistic health and wellness.

In essence, "Dark Calories and Toxic Oils Detox for Healthy Healing" encapsulates a journey of discovery and empowerment, offering readers the knowledge and tools needed to reclaim their health from the harmful effects of seed oils and vegetable oils. By adopting a mindful approach to nutrition, embracing natural healing practices, and fostering a holistic lifestyle, individuals can embark on a path towards vibrant health, longevity, and overall well-being.

APPENDICES

RESOURCES AND FURTHER READING

As you embark on your journey to detox from toxic oils and embrace a healthier lifestyle, expanding your knowledge through additional resources can be invaluable. The following list includes recommended books, articles, websites, and organizations that delve deeper into topics related to nutrition, detoxification, and holistic health.

Recommended Books

- **"Deep Nutrition: Why Your Genes Need Traditional Food"** by Catherine Shanahan Dr. Catherine Shanahan's groundbreaking exploration of the link between modern dietary

habits and chronic diseases provides a foundational understanding of nutrition's role in health.
- **"The Big Fat Surprise: Why Butter, Meat and Cheese Belong in a Healthy Diet"** by Nina Teicholz Nina Teicholz challenges conventional wisdom about dietary fats and presents compelling evidence supporting the health benefits of natural fats.
- **"In Defense of Food: An Eater's Manifesto"** by Michael Pollan Michael Pollan offers practical advice on how to navigate the confusing landscape of modern food choices and reclaim the joys of eating healthily.
- **"Eat to Beat Disease: The New Science of How Your Body Can Heal Itself"** by William W. Li This book explores the body's natural ability to heal and offers insights into foods that support immune function, reduce inflammation, and promote overall wellness.
- **"The Plant Paradox: The Hidden Dangers in 'Healthy' Foods That Cause Disease and Weight Gain"** by Steven R. Gundry Dr. Steven Gundry examines how certain plant-based foods may contribute to health issues and provides guidance on choosing healthier alternatives.

Recommended Articles

- Shanahan, C. (2020). *Vegetable oils, (Francis Marion Press)* An in-depth look at the

detrimental effects of vegetable oils on cellular health and overall well-being.
- Kummerow, F. (2013). *The negative effects of hydrogenated trans fats and what to do about it* Discusses the history and health implications of trans fats, advocating for their removal from the food supply.
- Mozaffarian, D., & Ludwig, D. S. (2010). *The 2010 dietary guidelines - the best recipe for health?* Analyzes the strengths and weaknesses of the 2010 dietary guidelines and proposes improvements based on current scientific evidence.

Useful Websites and Organizations

- **American Heart Association** Provides resources on heart-healthy eating, including guidelines on fats and oils. Website: www.heart.org
- **NutritionFacts.org** Offers evidence-based articles and videos on nutrition topics, including the effects of oils on health. Website: www.nutritionfacts.org
- **World Health Organization (WHO)** Publishes reports and guidelines on nutrition, including recommendations for reducing saturated and trans fats in the diet. Website: www.who.int/nutrition/en/
- **Environmental Working Group (EWG)** Provides consumer guides and resources on food

additives, pesticides, and sustainable food choices. Website: www.ewg.org
- **National Center for Complementary and Integrative Health (NCCIH)** Offers information on alternative therapies and integrative approaches to health and wellness. Website: www.nccih.nih.gov

GLOSSARY OF TERMS

1. **Seed Oils**: Oils extracted from the seeds of plants, often high in omega-6 fatty acids.
2. **Vegetable Oils**: Oils derived from various plants, including seeds, nuts, and fruits, used in cooking and food processing.
3. **Dark Calories**: Calories derived from unhealthy fats and oils that contribute to metabolic dysfunction and chronic disease.
4. **Chronic Inflammation**: Persistent inflammation in the body linked to various diseases such as cardiovascular disease and arthritis.
5. **Oxidative Stress**: Imbalance between free radicals and antioxidants in the body, leading to cell damage.
6. **Metabolic Disorders**: Conditions affecting metabolism, including diabetes, obesity, and metabolic syndrome.
7. **Mental Health**: Psychological well-being and cognitive function.
8. **Cognitive Function**: Mental processes involved in thinking, learning, and memory.
9. **Biochemistry**: Chemical processes and substances occurring within living organisms.
10. **Antioxidants**: Compounds that inhibit oxidation and neutralize free radicals.
11. **Omega-3 Fatty Acids**: Essential fatty acids found in fish and some plant sources, known for their anti-inflammatory properties.

12. **Omega-6 Fatty Acids**: Polyunsaturated fats found in vegetable oils, necessary in moderation but excessive intake can lead to inflammation.
13. **Inflammatory Response**: Immune system reaction to injury or infection, involving swelling, redness, and pain.
14. **Free Radicals**: Unstable molecules with unpaired electrons, causing oxidative damage to cells.
15. **Nutritional Epidemiology**: Study of dietary patterns and their impact on health outcomes in populations.
16. **Personalized Nutrition**: Tailoring dietary advice to individual genetic, metabolic, and health factors.
17. **Microbiome**: Microbial communities living in and on the human body, influencing health and digestion.
18. **Probiotics**: Live bacteria and yeasts beneficial for gut health when consumed in adequate amounts.
19. **Prebiotics**: Fiber-rich foods that promote the growth of beneficial gut bacteria.
20. **Functional Foods**: Foods enriched with nutrients or bioactive substances for health benefits beyond basic nutrition.
21. **Malnutrition**: Imbalance in nutrient intake, leading to undernutrition or overnutrition.
22. **Food Fortification**: Adding vitamins, minerals, or other nutrients to foods to address deficiencies.

23. **Sustainable Food Systems**: Practices that promote food production while minimizing environmental impact.
24. **Environmental Sustainability**: Meeting present needs without compromising the ability of future generations to meet theirs.
25. **Plant-Based Diet**: Emphasizing whole, plant foods while minimizing or excluding animal products.
26. **Holistic Health**: Approach considering physical, mental, emotional, and spiritual well-being.
27. **Stress Management**: Techniques to reduce and cope with stress, promoting overall health.
28. **Mindfulness**: Practice of being present and aware in the moment, reducing stress and improving focus.
29. **Dietary Guidelines**: Recommendations for healthy eating and nutrition based on scientific evidence.
30. **Public Health**: Discipline focused on improving health and preventing diseases in populations.
31. **Policy Change**: Systematic efforts to modify laws, regulations, or practices to achieve specific goals, such as improving food standards.
32. **Nutrient Density**: Ratio of nutrients to calories in a food, indicating its nutritional value.
33. **Food Security**: Access by all people at all times to enough food for an active, healthy life.
34. **Culinary Practices**: Traditional methods of food preparation and cooking techniques.

35. **Inflammation**: Body's immune response to injury, infection, or irritation, causing redness, swelling, and pain.
36. **Cardiovascular Disease**: Conditions affecting the heart and blood vessels, including heart attacks and strokes.
37. **Diabetes**: Chronic condition affecting blood sugar levels and insulin production or sensitivity.
38. **Obesity**: Condition of excessive body fat accumulation, leading to health problems.
39. **Cancer**: Disease characterized by abnormal cell growth with the potential to invade other tissues.
40. **Gut Health**: Balance of microorganisms and digestive processes in the gastrointestinal tract.
41. **Detoxification**: Process of removing toxins from the body, often supported through dietary and lifestyle changes.
42. **Wellness**: Active pursuit of activities, choices, and lifestyles that lead to a state of holistic health.
43. **Cellular Health**: Maintenance of cellular functions and structures essential for overall health.
44. **Rejuvenation**: Restoration of vitality, energy, and youthfulness.
45. **Mind-Body Connection**: Interaction between mental and physical health, influencing overall well-being.

46. **Environmental Impact**: Effect of human activities on the natural environment and ecosystems.
47. **Biodiversity**: Variety of life forms in a given ecosystem, contributing to ecological balance.
48. **Nutrient Absorption**: Process of absorbing nutrients from food into the bloodstream for use by cells.
49. **Epidemiology**: Study of patterns, causes, and effects of health and disease conditions in defined populations.
50. **Regulatory Measures**: Laws, policies, and regulations enacted to promote public health and safety.
51. **Sustainable Agriculture**: Farming practices that meet current food production needs without compromising future generations' ability to do so.
52. **Food Labeling**: Information displayed on food packaging about its nutritional content and ingredients.
53. **Bioavailability**: Proportion of a nutrient or substance that enters circulation when introduced into the body and is made available for biological processes.
54. **Dietary Fiber**: Non-digestible carbohydrates that promote digestive health and regular bowel movements.
55. **Caloric Intake**: Amount of energy derived from food and beverages consumed.

56. **Nutrient Deficiency**: Lack of essential vitamins, minerals, or other nutrients required for optimal health.
57. **Digestive Health**: Maintenance of healthy gastrointestinal function and nutrient absorption.
58. **Immune Function**: Body's ability to defend against pathogens and foreign substances.
59. **Food Allergies**: Adverse immune reactions to specific foods or ingredients.
60. **Food Sensitivities**: Non-allergic adverse reactions to certain foods, often involving digestive discomfort.
61. **Macronutrients**: Nutrients required in large amounts for energy production and bodily functions, including carbohydrates, proteins, and fats.
62. **Micronutrients**: Essential vitamins and minerals required in smaller amounts for various physiological processes.
63. **Amino Acids**: Building blocks of proteins essential for growth, repair, and maintenance of body tissues.
64. **Essential Fatty Acids**: Fats required for biological processes but not synthesized by the body, necessitating dietary intake.
65. **Insulin Resistance**: Condition in which cells become less responsive to the hormone insulin, leading to elevated blood sugar levels.
66. **Metabolic Syndrome**: Cluster of conditions—increased blood pressure, high blood sugar,

excess body fat around the waist, and abnormal cholesterol or triglyceride levels—that occur together, increasing the risk of heart disease, stroke, and diabetes.

67. **Hormonal Balance**: Equilibrium of hormones in the body necessary for optimal health and function.
68. **Endocrine Disruptors**: Chemical substances that interfere with the endocrine (hormonal) system, potentially causing adverse developmental, reproductive, neurological, and immune effects.
69. **Processed Foods**: Foods that have undergone mechanical or chemical alterations during manufacturing, often containing added sugars, fats, and preservatives.
70. **Whole Foods**: Foods that are minimally processed or refined and do not contain added ingredients, preserving their natural nutritional integrity.
71. **Vitamins**: Essential organic compounds required in small amounts for various metabolic processes, growth, and immunity.
72. **Minerals**: Inorganic substances essential for biological functions, such as bone health, nerve function, and energy metabolism.
73. **Phytonutrients**: Bioactive compounds found in plant-based foods that have health-promoting properties and antioxidant effects.

74. **Digestive Enzymes**: Proteins that facilitate the breakdown of food into smaller, absorbable nutrients during digestion.
75. **Anxiety**: Emotional state characterized by feelings of worry, fear, or unease, affecting mental well-being.
76. **Depression**: Mood disorder characterized by persistent sadness, loss of interest or pleasure in activities, and impaired daily functioning.
77. **Cognitive Decline**: Reduction in cognitive abilities, including memory, reasoning, and decision-making processes, often associated with aging or neurological conditions.
78. **Holistic Medicine**: Approach to healthcare that considers the whole person—body, mind, spirit, and emotions—in the prevention, diagnosis, and treatment of illness.
79. **Environmental Toxins**: Chemical or biological agents present in the environment that can harm human health through exposure via air, water, soil, or food.
80. **Inflammation Markers**: Biomarkers in the blood or tissues indicating the presence and extent of inflammation in the body.
81. **Pro-inflammatory Foods**: Foods that promote inflammation in the body, potentially exacerbating chronic conditions.
82. **Anti-inflammatory Foods**: Foods that help reduce inflammation and support overall health, including fruits, vegetables, and omega-3 fatty acids.

83. **Oxidative Damage**: Harmful effects caused by oxidative stress on cells, proteins, and DNA, contributing to aging and disease.
84. **Nutritional Supplements**: Products containing vitamins, minerals, herbs, amino acids, or other dietary substances intended to supplement the diet and support health.
85. **Food Additives**: Substances added to food during processing to improve taste, texture, appearance, or shelf life, including preservatives, colorings, and flavor enhancers

Made in the USA
Coppell, TX
18 July 2024